YIN
Is the New
BLACK

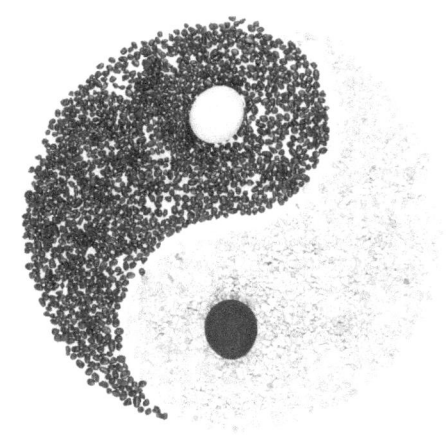

HOW TO GET RID *Of*
IMBALANCES IN YOUR LIFE

PETRA RAKEBRANDT

To contact the author, visit Website:
www.PetraRakebrandt.com and www.PetraMindBodyWork.com

ISBN-10: 1530995558
ISBN-13: 978-1530995554
Printed in the United States of America

Editor: Amanda Filippelli
Designer: Amie Olson
Photographer: Nathalie Colucci

To all the souls
who have touched my soul.

Contents

Acknowledgements

I would like to take the opportunity to send out my love and gratitude to everybody who's come into my life to make me a better person, who's helped me to be the person I am now, who's pushed me through and helped me in hard times. Without you, I would not be the teacher and healer that I am today.

Life is a journey that we cannot go alone. We need each other, and it is important that we support each other, acknowledge each other, respect each other. We are all different, and everybody has to find their own journey to follow. There is no right or wrong journey. There is only the one you are supposed to live. Seek it out and move along.

I was on a journey which was not wrong for me, but which didn't feel right. I always knew I'd have to change my path, but that is often difficult to do, and we resist the changes we need to make. But what you resist persists. Eventually, we meet people and we get into situations which help us. It is up to us to try and understand all the events and souls we encounter on our journey.

I thank you for all the support during different parts of my path, in my personal and professional life. I am so grateful for the teachers who helped me to heal. I believe if we heal our soul, we can heal others and change the world. I hope, from the depths of my heart, that this book will provide some help and healing for you.

LIFE IS A JOURNEY,
NOT A DESTINATION.

-SOUZA

Introduction

The fact that you have chosen this book may mean that you are looking for change—that deep inside you, you know that your life should be different. You know that you can improve your health, diet, and the way you exercise. You can improve the way you treat yourself. I am sure you have it within you to be able to change whatever is necessary. Just listen to your inner voice. Sit quietly and listen. When we listen on the inside and heal our souls, we can heal other souls around us. Through healing others, the universe will be a better place. But we have to start with ourselves. What's first on our journey? We have to start loving ourselves!

In 2003, I had a big change in my life. My husband and I decided to "break up" after more than a year of marriage coaching. I really needed to leave my job, which I thought was neither important for the world nor for my personal life. I needed to find the way of life that I had always longed for and dreamed of. How would I find this life? Why was I so unhappy all these thirty-five years of my life? Why was I sick most of the time with lingering sinus infections, toothaches, and back pain? I thought, *This can't be the way life is supposed to be.* I was always looking for improvement and happiness in shopping, in vacationing, in more studying, but none of this changed anything. I was always the same sad and sick person. Deep inside, I was sure there was a way to become happier and healthier. I had to realize that, as an individual, I have the power to change the direction of my life.

I was always interested in the soul. Just the word itself made me feel connected to something. It gave me a form of stability. I began coaching sessions with a life coach. My coach once said, "Ms. Rakebrandt, you have to start meditating to connect with your soul. You are an intuitive person. You will get all the answers. You are here for the search of your soul." These words made me so mad. Just hearing the word "meditating" made me angry. I was resistant to this view and thought, *Why does this person think it is okay to tell me what I should do?* Obviously, I had sought help when I took a coach. However, hearing the raw truth was too much.

Today, I know that my life coach pushed the right internal button in me. I was just afraid of starting on a path to inner connection with myself. I was scared of finding myself. I was scared of seeing the truth because the truth would be totally different from what I was thinking, feeling, and living up until then.

Until that point in my life, I had reached every goal that I set out to reach. I studied engineering and received a Master of Business Administration degree. I worked as a managing director and made a handsome income. I had a nice home and a "normal" marriage. Still, I was so unhappy. Something profound was missing. I hated my body. I hated the emptiness inside.

So the adventure began…

According to Buddhism, living your dharma means to live in conformity with your nature and duty. I wish I had known what my dharma was. The purpose to my life was completely lost. Something had to change. That way of living involved being in the office from 9am-7pm most days. Then, I would run to the gym and be back home around 10pm for dinner or just snacking. I would watch television and then fall to sleep. *Is this it?* I thought. No way. *What's the point?*

I believe that we, as human beings, are pretty weak. We only change when something bad happens—disease, a catastrophic situation, an accident, the death of a loved one, a divorce. These are moments when we can develop strength, when we see through and are able to change. Why is it so difficult to look, think, and analyze before things get really bad? Why is it difficult to identify something that needs changed?

In my own experience, I suffered a long time. I felt unhappy and I wanted to change, but only when the pain got worse, once I was having more sleepless nights, and back pain that would not go away, only then did I start to get active. Before that, I just ignored it, pushed it away, and hoped that it would get better by just waiting. If we do this in business, ignore processes that are not working, the business will "die" soon. The business world cannot wait that long. A company does inventory once a year to analyze assets and overages. So if companies take the time for due diligence, why are we not checking in on our lives and relationships regularly? Why are we not giving ourselves a chance to understand or realize if something is on the wrong track, or if something could be improved?

By checking in, for example, in our relationships, we can analyze the quality time we spend with our partner, and either we find out we're spending a great deal of quality time together or we might identify the need to implement changes, to set dates with our partner, so that we don't completely slip apart. Why do we not regularly examine where we are at in life? Is it just fear? Why do we not consider where we are and where we want to be? Maybe a makeover or a reset is needed? Are we already afraid of what it could mean or of finding out that something is off? Is that the reason we wait for the challenge or the shock, which pushes us to the edge where we have to react?

Speaking for myself in retrospect, it was mostly fear. I didn't know what to do or why I was unhappy. *Where should I start to change? And how? And what?* I also felt fear around how to explain my feelings to other people—my parents, colleagues, friends.

When my husband and I decided to stop living in our "sad relationship," it woke me up. Now was the time to go deeper. I was at the edge. At this moment, I had the courage to do it all. I could change my life. I could wake up and start over. Something had obviously been missing inside of me for a long time, and I really wanted to find out what it was.

Changing your life, believe me, is not always the easiest task. First, you have to know what to change, then where and how to change it. I was not even sure what my problem was. I just felt empty. I felt like I was in the wrong place, maybe even in the wrong body. I always had the feeling that I was born in the wrong family, and I had no goal in life. I needed to reset the whole system. *But how?*

I was sure that I was burning out. We had been having a lot of trouble in the office for at least two years. At the same time, my relationship was not functioning. I felt out of control. No wonder that the body begins to try to communicate this to you. The body's way of sharing this with you is through pain—everything from sleeping problems and digestive problems to infections. So often we do not want to listen to our body's language. We ignore the signs from our body. I believe this is especially true if you are a strong willed person like I am. I do not let my body take over through pain or sickness. Even if my body is showing me pain, I control it. I take a pain killer and keep going. "I am strong. I can manage. My pain is not putting me down." Yes, that is what we believe, but only up to a certain point, until our bodies react to this approach and another pain or symptom shows up. And so it becomes a continuous cycle.

The more we try to cover up symptoms, the more we suffer. We need to work to find the courage to try and find out the real problem instead of taking care of just the symptoms. I see it in my work every day. Before people start to face the real problem, they try to cure just the symptoms rather than seek out the root cause of the symptoms. I did this for many years. I treated my back pain with massages and physiotherapy, and to treat my toothaches, I ran to the dentist once a month, but he could not find anything. I took medication for my stomach and digestion problems, but nothing really changed anything.

I got to the point where I had no other solution than to stop it all. I think that my subconscious mind had known for a long time what to do. I had known for years that I was not living the life I wanted to live, and that's what was causing all of my physical problems. But my conscious mind tried to avoid recognizing it, until I surrendered and gave up and let my subconscious mind take over. This is where yoga and meditation helped.

When I started to sit down and really listen to what was stored in my subconscious mind, I understood what I wanted and needed. The conscious mind is so rational and wants to make all the decisions from a rational, calculated point of view—salary and safety play bigger roles than happiness. Of course, it is scary in the beginning to think that you need to change to be happier because you are used to a nice salary and fear is coming up around how to provide and continue living the life you are used to!

My view now, based on the knowledge I have gained in the last ten years, is that the first thirty-five years of my life was filled with YANG elements—stress, fast energy, running, jumping, biking, huffing and puffing. The people around me were also full of yang energy. They were stressed and complaining. Their days were filled with tasks and errands. Of course, I filled my body with yang food like coffee, meat, processed food, eggs, sugar, sugar, (and more sugar), spicy food, and salty food. I could not get enough of it. Sometimes, while driving home after work, I'd eat a bag of sugary junk food. As soon as I came in the house, I "balanced" it out with a bag of potato chips. I needed salt after the bag of sugar! This is what I did to feel calm and okay. Yes, I felt calm and okay, but not happy and healthy!

Sometimes, I went straight from the office to the gym for a ninety-minute spinning class to get that angry and choleric energy out of my body. I just had to move and scream to get rid of the stress. Of course, a yoga class would have killed me at that point. At one point in my life, I gave it a chance, but I could not handle it. Being quiet in a yoga pose made me understand that I had to face my situation. No, I was not ready. So I continued to stay in this yang energy, piling more on top and telling myself that I was in control of the situation. "It is my life, and I am in charge."

After spinning, I sat down in the sauna and my mind became quiet for fifteen to twenty minutes. These were the moments when I heard an inner voice, "Petra, how long do you want to go on like this?" Then, I felt this deep sadness inside. It felt like a very sad child was talking to me. I saw myself looking at this sad child with sorrow and pity, not knowing what to do. I told myself, "Stay in there. One day, everything will be okay. For now, all is okay as well. Great job. You have time to do sports and time to hang in the sauna." With these thoughts, I went home, went to bed, and convinced myself all was good and that it would change one day.

Chapter 1

The Yin and the Yang Systems

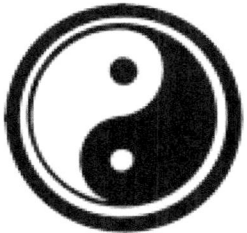

We all know the symbol of yin and yang. I remember when the symbol meant something cool in my teenage years. Suddenly, everybody had it on bracelets, on t-shirts, or on bags. The most "courageous" people got a tattoo of the symbol. I remember wondering what the symbol was all about. I never thought that it would become such a guiding symbol for me later in life.

Yin is the black side with the white dot in it. Yang is the white side with the black dot in it. The relationship between yin and yang is often described in terms of sunlight moving over a mountain and a valley. Yin, which literally means the "shady place" or "north slope," and equal to the moon, is the dark area occluded by the mountain's bulk. Likewise, yang literally means the "sunny place" or "south slope," and represents the sun. Yang is the brightly lit portion. That is easy to understand as the sun is coming from the south. So, it is shining at the south side of the hill and on the north side of the river. That's why the north side of the river is yang. As the sun moves across the sky, yin and yang gradually trade places with each other, revealing what was obscured and obscuring what was revealed.

According to Chinese theory, yin and yang are two forces in the universe. Yin is the passive and negative force. Yang is the active, positive force. According to this theory, wise people will detect these forces in the seasons, in their food, and so on, and will regulate their lives accordingly.

Characteristics of yin and yang are:

yin	yang
slow	fast
soft	hard
diffuse	solid
cold	hot
wet	dry
passive	aggressive
water	fire
earth	sky
moon	sun
femininity	masculinity
night time	day time

Image Source: Osgood, Charles E. "From Yang and Yin To and Or but." Language 49.2 (1973): 380–412, JSTOR. 16 November 2008, jstor.org

As you can see in the table, the yin and yang model shows duality. We see opposites as well as the complementary aspects of each. With both sides, we get balance. There is no judgement in the characteristics of yin and yang. One is not better than the other. We need both to gain balance. For example, according to nature, a woman is more soft and receptive. If she is giving too much or getting too strong, even more masculine, her nature will be in imbalance and she might get stressed out, overwhelmed, or even sick. In a relationship, it could bring imbalance if the woman is acting like a man. A power struggle can occur and the man might lose his place in the relationship. On the other hand, if a man gets too soft or too feminine, his nature is out of balance as well. Please do not judge the characteristics. As I said, we need both.

When we look at the characteristics of yin and yang, some of them seem to be more positive or negative. We might think the characteristic of light is more positive than the characteristic of dark, but again, the system will show us that we need to acknowledge both for balance. Of course, we have a light side in us, which gives us a sense of positivity, and we try to hide our dark side, which is there as well, whether we believe in it or not. But we often try to hide this dark side because we interpret it as negative, and by doing so, we get out of balance. Take, for example, the sun moving over the mountain. The sun is light, but at the same time, it is creating shadow—something dark. Often, we do not want to see this dark side in us because the dark side could be the anger we are carrying, fears, regrets, or resentments. If we try to avoid all of these feelings, we get out of balance.

In Chinese philosophy and traditional Chinese medicine, this is exactly what is described—that all of these dualities are necessary and complimentary. If one quality is considered deficient, imbalance will occur. And if you look in nature, it is impossible that one of the dual aspects would disappear. For example, there cannot always be day or night. There cannot always be heat or coldness. These characteristic are interdependent and both necessary for balance in nature, and we are part of nature.

We can alleviate ourselves of a lot of stress if we understand and start acknowledging imbalances in our lives. To do so, we need to acknowledge the positive and negative parts of us and in us.

Look at yourself for a minute and examine what you do normally. Are you able to see all of your "positive" traits? Or do you like to beat yourself up all the time and see more of the negative? Doing so causes emotional imbalances. There is another segment of people who always see just the positive parts, which is not balancing either. Remember the yin and yang symbol—where there is a yin, there is a yang, and where there is a yang, there is a yin. The system is only in balance when all forces are complementary. Even if you try to avoid or hide some aspect, nature will bring it up through situations, pain, relationships, you name it.

Start reflecting on your life where you feel balanced right now and where you would like to find more balance. Look for parts in your life where you are hiding something—an emotion or desire. Look for why you hide it, what is the cost of hiding it, and what would happen if you let it show up?

When I look back now, I realize that I was very unhappy and out of balance as I was hiding many parts of myself. I was not living my life and I just tried to live according to what I thought was expected of me. That cannot at all be a balanced life.

In this book, I do not want to talk too much about the history of yin and yang. Merely, I just want to mention that it is an ancient idea. I recommend you read further about it, get more familiar with it, and especially come to understand why it's important to find balance.

The yin and yang system can be applied to everything in our lives—to our bodies, our work, the way we exercise, our relationships, nutrition and the way we eat. Actually, we can apply it to the way we live and even the way we love.

We can also apply yin and yang balance to our food. While there are many historical and modern schools of Daoism with different teachings on the subject, many Taoists regard their diet as extremely important to their physical, mental, and spiritual health. Diet connects to the amount of qi, or energy, we consume.

Some early Daoist diets called for bigu, meaning "avoiding grains," based on the belief that immortality could be achieved in this way. The ancient Taoist texts of the Taiping Jing suggest that individuals who attained the state of complete ziran would not need food at all, but could instead sustain themselves by absorbing the cosmic qi.

But food is the energy our bodies run on and we can easily get out of balance by eating the wrong food or by eating too much processed food. In our society, we are under constant pressure, and we do not take enough time for proper meals, made with well-chosen ingredients and love at home. Because we also suffer under the lack of time to grocery shop, we end up with fast food and processed food, which is mostly too salty or too sweet, keeping our whole body system in imbalance.

Everything in life is energy, so start to see your life more like energy flowing everywhere. When you get in touch with your own energy, learn how to use energy and to feel energy, then it gets easier to find balance.

The foundation of traditional Chinese medicine attempts to create as much possible balance between the two energetic polarities, to hopefully establish homoeostasis within the mind, body, and spirit. We achieve homoeostasis when we direct our everyday lifestyle choices to level out these two polar opposites.

On a daily basis, we should be trying to counter our yin and yang actions. If you're mentally challenging yourself on a busy day, be sure to counter yang energy with a physically restful and restorative yin action, like gentle yoga. By doing this, you counter the mental yang energy with a corresponding physical activity, balancing out the demanding yang with nourishing yin.

When I reflect back on my office life—sitting there for about eight hours, being on the phone, then in meetings, doing calculations in between, having two or three coffees, then sitting on the full subway— all of those things represent a lot of yang energy. In the evening, during my ninety minutes of spinning at the gym, there was noisy music with screaming and yelling. I was sweating with a high heart rate and unaware that I was putting more yang energy on my body. Day-in and day-out, it was like that. In retrospect, I wonder how I wasn't more sick! Why do we put so much pressure on ourselves and on our bodies? Why do we treat our bodies and minds like that? There cannot be any self-love when we do this.

In my personal example, I think I denied myself completely. I denied my desires. I denied my dreams. I denied my body. Looking back, it feels as if I punished my body for something. I was mean to myself, there was no self-love at all, and I guess, at that time, I did not even know what self-love was. The reason for that could be that we never properly learn what self-love is and that we have the right to take care of our bodies and minds. We are mostly educated to look at how we fit into the system, how we can please others first instead of doing right by ourselves. If you want to find balance in your life, I recommend that you start observing your actions more, as well as your thoughts and desires, so that you can even out your actions in the pursuit of a yin and yang life.

You always want to stay balanced, right at your center of gravity. And if we are centered, we can make better decisions, we know what we want and what is good for us. Only if you are connected to yourself and in your center, can you listen to your intuition.

Try and imagine your life, your actions, feelings, and thoughts are governed by a scale balancing the yin and yang energies within your mind and body. I am sure that if you work for years on yang energy, your body will find a reason to bring balance in. You can even interpret a heart attack as a means to bring your body down, to give you rest, to force you, as nature needs and wants to be balanced. After day, there is night, and there is day again, and so forth. Nature always looks for balance. We become depleted when we just focus on one area of our lives, so start practicing and exercising yin and yang polarities in all areas of your life. Do it consciously. Do not wait until something happens that forces you. When you have both yin and yang in balance, you are aligned and centered.

Chapter 2

Changes for a Balanced Life

When I reached the point that I needed to make changes in my life, I had no idea where to start. I did not even know what was wrong in my life. I knew that I wanted to feel better, to be happier, to feel more energized, and to have a smile on my face every day. I'd had enough of complaining and listening to the complaints of others around me. I wanted to have a different body. I wanted more fun at work. I wanted to eat healthier, and I desired a relationship that could fulfill me on all levels. So many things, but where to start?

I needed a coach, and I really value the work of life coaches. My husband and I had picked a person for couples coaching because we understood we couldn't balance our love life without help. What we came to understand, though, is that we could not just light up one section of our life. Everything is connected, and if you are unhappy in your job, it affects your relationship, and if you have problems with your partner, it can affect some other area in your life. I was starting to see how different aspects of my life were indicating imbalance in my relationship.

For example, food is a great indicator if your life is in balance or not. If you use food other than to nurture your body, you can be sure that areas of your life are not balanced and that you are compensating with food. Work is another indicator of your life balance. If you find yourself working extra hours to avoid being home, or if you work extra hours to avoid feeling lonely, your life is likely out of balance.

I really felt relieved when we started the coaching sessions. For the first time in many years, I felt there was a solution, and that a change for a happier life was possible. I was sure that I had found the right person to help me come out of my shell and try to find light in life. With her, I understood all the connections between different areas in my life—reasons why I could not be happy and why my husband could not be happy. Sometimes, I was angry with her, especially each time that she mentioned, over and over again, in a very loving way of course, that I should start meditation. I got mad because, deep inside, I must have known that she was right. At that time though, this step was just too much. I know today that I had so much fear of what I would discover in meditation about myself, about my family, and my beliefs. It was just so scary that I wasn't ready to do it yet.

Sometimes, small changes are already enough to get better results in life. For some people, just starting to eat healthier, like adding in more vegetables, can be enough. Or, alternatively, quitting the glass of alcohol after work can do a lot for a person's health and diet.

About alcohol. I once had a client who lost all of her excessive weight by quitting the daily two to three glasses of alcohol in the evening as stress relief after work. Instead, she instituted a balanced workout two times a week. While these changes may be easy for some, they can be very difficult for others. Some people need bigger changes. An apple a day would not do it for them. Maybe a break up, a career change, or even the move to a different city might be necessary. The goal is to find your own balance.

I guess everybody can relate when I say that the most difficult thing in life is figuring out what you want! And this applies to all areas of life—what kind of job you want, what city you want to live in, who your partner should be, whether you even want to be in a relationship, or sometimes it is just knowing if you want to eat pizza or salad. We face decisions every day, and some are easy, and some are not. And again, here, I want to mention that it is necessary to know your own center, to know who you are, to be connected with your Self in order to make the right decisions. We can only be connected with our Self when we are in balance—only from that point can we connect to our intuition and be sure about what we want.

Decisions are often made out of fear, which is not the best place to make them from. I did not change anything earlier in my life because of fear—fear of not knowing what is coming, the fear of how to earn money, the fear of telling people that I want to be separated from my husband, the fear of my boss when quitting my job. Fear was my motivation to stay in that mess for so long and to accept pain for so long, not understanding that I am causing even more pain to myself and probably to others.

In regards to the yin and yang system, fear is as much a part of life as is joy. So, by just not looking at fear, it is impossible to find balance. Fear really gave me the sensation of being out of control, and when you feel out of control, you feel weak, sensitive, in danger maybe, not at all empowered, and not at all in balance! So, believe me, the moment I started working with my coach who made me look at all the dark sides, like fear and negative emotions such as guilt, I already gained a bit more control and connection with myself. I found greater understanding about my situation and more trust and faith in the direction of change, that change is possible, that balance is possible, and that pain can be avoided.

What often hinders us in finding balance and connection to ourselves is the idea that we all have to fit into a scheme—that there is one right way to follow to be a good person, to do things right, to be worthy. That is wrong. We are all different, and we have the right to be different. We have different interests, we have different preferences, we have different opinions.

Our differences define our bio-individuality. There is no diet that works for everybody in the same way. What is good for me might be poison for somebody else (just think of allergies). To find balance and get rid of imbalances, you have to be conscious and attentive, looking at your diet and what makes you feel good or bad, what makes you feel bloated or even gives you headaches or digestive problems. You have to garner a general understanding of the functioning of the body.

I am sorry to tell you that there was never, ever a diet that was going to work perfectly for you in the long run. Going on a diet for two weeks is simple. It will probably bring short term changes. You might even lose weight. However, if you fall back into your old habits, those two weeks are just two weeks where you did something different. You will not experience the long term results you were hoping for. Dieting is like treating the symptom instead of the root cause.

People who come to me for coaching because they feel unhealthy in their body and unhappy in life mostly think they need to lose weight. But often, they do not need a diet. They need to find balance through a lifestyle change—sometimes even just a change of thoughts.

To do this, you have to understand what is going on in your life and in your mind. Do not believe all of what you think every day! We are all trained and conditioned in a certain way how and what to think.

It starts in childhood. We watch what our parents do, they tell us what they think, we believe them, and we make their thoughts and beliefs our thoughts and beliefs. These are now our programs for life. Some stuff gets added on in school and in our careers—we get programmed by teachers, then in jobs. Everything that happens to us trains and programs our brains.

If we do not question these thought and belief systems, we just follow them blindly, passing them onto our children. That's how history repeats itself in families. It is in our subconscious minds, in our cells. It becomes so "normal," like driving a car. You don't need to think about when to push the pedal to change gear; your body is doing it automatically—the same way you repeat your thoughts.

But if some programs are not working for you because your nature is different, because your dreams and desires are totally different from what you were told to want, because your purpose in life is different than what you were trained for, you will feel out of your center, not connected, and something in your body and mind will start feeling confused and out of balance. That is the starting point. There are so many beliefs about food, body image, beliefs around money, marriage, you name it, and it is all of those beliefs that throw us out of balance.

If you think and believe all day, "I never lose weight," then you program your body to not lose weight. Everything is anchored deep down in our subconsciousness. As long as you choose not to explore and find out what's behind this, how it is serving you to believe it, finding out what is hidden, and what is blocking your clarity, then you will have to work really hard to make changes in your weight. And this is the same with relationships, with work, with your whole concept of the world.

Changes can be made by examining your emotions. Look and observe your emotions. This is not easy in the beginning, because often, we are taught to not evaluate our emotions. We are even taught that we cannot trust our emotions. We are told to stop crying. We are told that injuries aren't that bad and that your knee does not really hurt from falling down. You all can recall that situation from childhood. When you fell down as a kid, an adult would tell you that all is good. You may have known at the time it was not true. You may have felt that it hurts. You may have thought, *I feel stupid because I fell*. So, by getting told, "Stop, it is not so bad," you started thinking that maybe you were wrong for what you felt.

We have to analyze how we feel, why we feel the way we do, and how we would like to feel. Uncovering the reasons for why we feel like we feel can be very hurtful. It might be a situation from your childhood where you really suffered, but again, were told to forget. We have all these feelings buried in our cells, and one day, they pop out in the form of negative emotions like anger, or they manifest in bodily ways such as migraines, lower back pain, shoulder pain, or worse.

When it comes to food, most people are looking for the quick fix, a ten-day diet, or even better, a two-day diet, or a pill that will fix it, like a painkiller. Most people desire something that is fast and quick, something that requires no effort, something that is magic. In healing and finding balance in life, there is no such thing. If you take the time, and have the willpower and desire to really want to change something for the long term, it feels like magic. Life becomes magic when you finally live the life you want, love, and deserve.

A major healing is necessary. Only when we figure out what is wrong and what we want to change, can we change. Emotional healing and soul healing are the only things that can bring us back on track to a great life. It means facing what's happened in our lives, and letting ourselves experience a necessary emotional evolution. It is hard, but it is worth it.

When I look back at my life changes, I managed to find the job I love and to live in the place where I always wanted to be with a white sandy beach and sunshine. I have great relationships. I eat fresh and healthy food, and my lifestyle allows me to take care of myself every day. Was it easy to get here? No. A lot of crying was involved! Was it done overnight? No. It took years, and I think it is an ongoing process. I adjust each day as I learn more about myself, and I can understand it all more easily now. Now that I am closer to my center, to "my Self," after I analyzed what I really want, I am more at peace and able to make decisions from a place of balance. Taking care of myself is the priority now.

My work does not feel like work anymore. It is my passion, and I do it whenever I want to. I often organize retreats or workshops on weekends. Each time, I think, *If my boss, while I was an engineer, had called me into the office on a Sunday, I would have been so mad!!* Now, I "work" whenever I want, be it weekends or evenings. It is what I have chosen and what I like.

If you do something for eight hours a day and you do not like it, you will surely be imbalanced in body, mind, and spirit. You will feel so sluggish that you are not in the mood to exercise, not in the mood to cook a healthy meal, and not in the mood to cuddle with a loved one. Over time, your whole life becomes affected by the negative energy surrounding your work, and it will creep into each corner of your life, making finding balance more and more difficult.

I recommend that you take a minute to think where you could or would like to make changes to improve your life, lifestyle, and hence, your health and happiness. Just to give you an idea, for me, the main areas in life are:

- Relationship

- Exercise

- Food

- Work

- Sleep

We need to regularly examine these five areas of our lives. If life sucks in these areas and you are unhappy, then you have a lot of imbalances in your life. If you make changes here (sometimes only tiny changes are necessary), you will soon feel happier, more energized, more connected to yourself, and more in union with your SELF. You also will be able to improve the life of people around you, from your family and friends to your workplace and beyond. So, if you start with yourself, it will have a much bigger impact than you think. You can help others to change their lives through your example.

Chapter 3

How I
Found Balance

There was a time when my life almost completely fell apart. The night before I started my new position as managing director was the night my husband and I decided to break up. What a moment! Of course, that was not the day where I could go to work and be heartbroken. So, I kept smiling. I did not want that situation to influence my work life. So, I kept it a secret. At work, they thought my private life was fine. For me, that felt like it was the best decision, but playing a role you cannot identify with makes your heart and soul ache. My husband and I talked about divorce for a long time, so it was not as big and sad or horrible of a moment for me. It was just making the decision; we were almost separated long before that. Of course, no matter what, it hurt.

This is where I learned how important it is to be strong, but also to be honest with yourself. Facing problems and making decisions are the most important things if you want to improve something.

Facing the problem? Yes, that's what's necessary. I never liked people in my jobs who complained about their situation but never changed anything. Once, in my first job as a technical drawer, I had a colleague who seemed to come to work just to complain and whine about life. Financially, she really did not have the need to go to work or to do the job she was doing, which she obviously absolutely hated. Still, she came and complained for at least five hours a day! Why? People, please, if you are feeling negative, please do not spread your negative energy everywhere and drain other people who might like the workplace. On the other hand, I probably have to thank her for showing me how hard it must be to do something that you really do not like. So, if you are in that position, I really recommend stepping up and taking responsibility. Either find things you like about your job or change your situation.

"People are always blaming their circumstances for what they are.
I don't believe in circumstances.
The people who get on in this world are the people who
get up and look for the circumstances they want,
and if they can't find them, make them."

-George Bernard Shaw, *Mrs. Warren's Profession*

I think that if I had not changed my relationship situation with my ex-husband, I might be more sick or even dead by now. Unhappiness cannot breed a healthy body and mind. I see it in my coaching practice that many illnesses like headaches, skin reactions, insomnia, etc. are psychosomatic, stress related, and situation related. There is no pill which can cure this.

The way my ex-husband and I managed our problems is, for me, the best way. We never blamed each other. We never accused each other. We just faced the situation that we were both unhappy. So, we asked ourselves, *Why stay in this and be unhappy for the rest of our lives?* (And, of course, our coach helped us to see it like this.)

We can always find reasons to remain in a current, even unhappy situation: We have a mortgage. We have kids. I also had simple thoughts like, *What about the apartment? How do we split things? Who gets what?* Or, *Soon it'll be Christmas and I do not want to be alone.* Or, *Being single again means that I am not worthy. I feel ashamed.* The worst thought for me at that time was that I could get sick, really sick, maybe a cancer, and that I would die alone. I think you get my point.

All of these thoughts just created fear, and fear became the motivation to stay in that unhappy place because things could be worse. But "this could be worse" is a construct of the mind. Again, it is in our subconsciousness and coming up to hinder us from doing what needs to be done to be in balance, to be who we want to be.

So instead of focusing on the fear, we have to look at the emotions that we would like to feel, at the things we would like to have in life. Regarding our relationships, questions like, "Do I still love this person?" and, "Do I feel loved?" or, "Does this relationship make me happy?" are more important to consider than the fears we have.

Luckily, I understood that I had to overcome my fear—the fear of being alone, of not managing something in the house, the fear of what other people will think. Everything until then was fear driven. Finally, through strength, courage, willpower to be happy, and being fed up with pain and daily complaints, I was pushed in the direction to face the real situation and to get out of it.

I often hear people saying that they stay together because there are kids involved. I can understand this, but sometimes, staying together is not the best for your children anyway. Unfortunately, I see too often in my clients that this decision is not the best option. The kids feel how unhappy everybody is with the situation, and what we teach kids with this behavior is to not face their problems. I am not judging these decisions, but in some cases, the fear of hurting our children is an excuse for not facing our problems, not facing the fear.

"A fear of weakness only strengthens weakness."

-Criss Jami, *Salomé: In Every Inch, In Every Mile*

My first step in facing my fear was to separate from my husband, and then I managed to get out of my job. I wanted to finish a project before I left, so it took me a while to get out, but finally, I was free to start healing my body, mind, and soul. I improved my life with yoga, meditation, massages, through detoxifying my body and digestive system, and through training for what I really loved—fitness, Pilates, and yoga. I even took the time to learn French. Through these actions, I brought balance back to my life by offsetting the overwhelming amount of yang energy with an abundance of yin.

Chapter 4

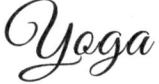

Yin and yang yoga are two different approaches and two different energies, but both energies are needed because they complement each other. Yang energy is more active, a fiery energy, which drives a person more than yin energy can. It drives and motivates all of your decisions emotionally, physically, and spiritually. To have balance, though, we need yin energy too, which is more restorative.

Yin energy allows the body to relax and slow down. Where yang is active energy, yin is resting energy. Through rest, our bodies get the chance to recover and nourish our cells. Elements of our body that are effected by yin energy are our body fluids, like the lymphatic system, water, and blood. Do not forget we are more than seventy percent water. Sleep, focus, and concentration, as well as determination are all affected and driven by yin energy too. But it does not stop there. Yin also influences our thoughts, beliefs, and values, even our purpose in life. So it is important for us to move our bodies within a balance of yin and yang yoga.

Without enough movement, we get stiff, our bodies get rusty, literally. The range of motion in our joints decreases, and on top of that, we store negative energy, which makes our bodies contract. We eat too much acidic food, which gets blocked in the cells and joints, and again, the body contracts, holding onto the excess acidity.

So isn't that enough reason to bring some yoga into your life so that you will become more flexible? Yoga will not only help your body to become more flexible, but also your mind. It will open you up and help you to try new things, because in yoga class, you see and learn that you have reserves in your body, that you can go deeper. Why not bring these lessons from the mat into your life? Why not try something new?

These days, yoga is quite a business in the Western world. I am not so sure how much it really has to do with Hindu spirituality or ascetic discipline. In this discipline, breath control, simple meditation, and the adoption of specific bodily postures is widely practiced for health and relaxation. Today, yoga often looks like acrobatic exercises. We have to take care that we do not bring our Western ego and passion for competition into yoga. Conversely, a major reason for implementing yoga in our lives is to overcome ego and negative emotions like jealousy, anger, or hate.

As it is said in the Bagavat Gita:

There, having the mind actively focused upon a single point,
with thought and sense activity controlled,
Sitting on a seat, one should practice yoga
for purification of the self.
With an aligned body, head, and neck—
keeping these steady, without movement;
Focusing the vision toward the tip of one's nose
without looking about in any direction.

-Bhagavad Gita, 6.12 - 13

For me, the sense I get from practicing yoga, asanas, pranayama, and meditation is that we can develop a fire, or a heat, inside. We can have a burning desire to better ourselves. In yoga, it is called TAPAS-heat, and when we use this heat, we motivate ourselves to grow and become better. We become aware of our drive, our motivation, our heat.

Another book, the Svetasvatara Upanishad, written in 600-500 BCE, explains the effects of the fire for one who is steeped in the practice of yoga:

When the fivefold qualities of yoga consisting of
the earth, water, fire, air and ether are firmly established
in the body, then in that body strengthened by the fire of yoga,
there is no place for sickness, old age and death.

-Svetasvatara Upanishad, 2.12

How can we use the text from the Svetasvatara Upanishad? It may mean making a change to certain habits. Heat can be produced by lowering and burning calories. It can eliminate negative addictions. It means we can improve oneself! We must connect with ourselves to be the best we can be!

Just by reading these two phrases from old literature, we can understand how important yoga should or could be in our lives. Only when we observe ourselves, can we purify ourselves and heal. What is more important than that? Isn't it getting more and more important in our society to bring balance into our lives and to get rid of imbalances? And what if it could be easy to do so with some yoga moves? Why not implement yoga and use it to improve different areas of your life? As all is connected, I promise that you will find more balance not just in your body, but also in your mind, your work, your relationships, and wherever you might feel stuck. As they say: Open hips, open mind!

I was lucky that a friend asked me to try her Hatha yoga class. She promised me that I would like it. So, I gave it another shot after my first horrible experience a few years before. This time, I loved it. Oh my god, what an experience! I felt my body. I felt being in my body. I felt I could work with my body. I loved the asanas (postures), which were kind of physically challenging. It gave me a totally new sense of myself and of my life. It gave me hope that all would be fine. I cannot even tell you why. I just felt so good.

I felt that I had found myself again, and at the same time, I was getting a good workout. I was sweating like I was on a thirty-minute run. I felt exhausted and relaxed at the same time. It was like traveling to a different place; a place you see for the first time, and you are just surprised because you never imagined something like that.

Of course, at that time, I was already in a different place than two years before when I had my first unpleasant experience with yoga. I finally felt ready and open to face whatever might come up from my deepest places inside—from my heart or soul.

I'd now experienced yang yoga. It was a real workout and the connection that I made with my spirit and mind was really amazing. Through the years, I learned how to connect to my body through yoga, and how to accept it, how to use it, how to make the best out of it, how to deal with challenges, how to overcome my ego, how to let go, how to challenge myself, and how to understand my limits. This is an ongoing process.

Until that yoga class, I participated in a lot of different sports, but this was a totally different experience of exercise. All the activities I had done before were active—the running, spinning, judo (fighting), or handball—were all super aggressive on my body. With yoga, I really get a different sense. I am challenging my body in poses like you challenge your body on a run, but because you are not moving, you get to the point and you have to observe your thoughts, your feelings, and your body. While running or biking, you are more concentrated on the function itself, the strength it takes, your heartbeat, and you probably have to fight with your will to keep going. But yoga is deeper; it gets to what is inside. While standing or laying in a pose, you start becoming aware, you start observing what was hidden until now, you shed light on it, you face it, and in the long run, accept it. By doing this, you find balance.

Chapter 5

Meditation

*"Meditation brings wisdom; lack of meditation leaves ignorance.
Know well what leads you forward and what holds you back,
and choose the path that leads to wisdom."*

-Buddha

When life feels unclear, when we feel lost, when we do not know what to do, and when we do not get enough sleep, there is imbalance in our lives. To help identify and remedy imbalance, meditation is another very important tool. When my coach told me to start meditation, especially as she had understood that I am a highly sensitive and spiritual person, I could not understand why she wanted me to do it. Today, I often see it in my clients' faces that they are surprised when I advise them to meditate. I probably made the same face years ago in front of my coach. And most people tell me they do not know how to meditate, or that they don't know how to control their thoughts.

What if I told you that meditation means that you make room for personal time to reflect and truly enjoy your life? Practice meditation, practice prayer, and connect with nature. Could you do that?

Of course, there is more to it, but to start, all you have to do is to learn how to become quiet and observe your breath and mind. Because many imbalances are just made up in our minds, we get a lot of information every day, have many details to think about, and in our brain, it is just too much to process. It can also be too much for our nervous system to process, so the easiest thing to do is just to sit down and try to stop your thoughts. Yes, I know, it isn't easy! But with some practice, I swear, if you can start just with a few minutes a day, your mind will become more quiet, it will become still, and you will have the chance to see what's going on deeper inside.

Being quiet gives us the chance to understand our inner self and to get a better understanding of our life's purpose. From this point, we are able to make better decisions—decisions that come from our deepest space. And again, it is this connection with our Self that helps us to find balance.

Many different institutions have done research on yoga and meditation and there is proof that both have an impact on different body functions and diseases. Both play a role on improving mood, reducing stress, decreasing blood pressure and heart rate, increasing lung capacity, and alleviating depression, anxiety, and insomnia. Meditation brings yin energy into your life so that you can restore some of your body functions that may be suffering from too much yang energy (from things like stress or extreme situations where your nervous system does not understand when a fight or flight situation is over).

Our fight or flight response is one of the most important systems in our body. It helped us to survive when we lived in the forest and were attacked by dangerous animals. Today, the dangerous animal has a different form—it can be a boss, a wife or husband, a friend. So our fight or flight system is always running on high, which means that stress hormones are being produced nonstop because we run from one stressful situation into another, making it difficult for our bodies to understand when to calm down.

A sequence of hormonal changes and psychological responses activate to help make fight or flight decisions when our bodies perceive danger. For our ancestors, it was super important to have this system working in case of a predator, but unfortunately, our bodies show the same reaction to stressors that are not life threatening—like a traffic jam, work pressure, or difficulty in a relationship with a partner. The fight or flight system is important, but research has shown that there are long-term effects on our bodies from continuous stress, like high blood pressure, insomnia, depression, anxiety, digestive problems, migraines, and back pain.

Meditation offers us a way to reclaim our bodies response systems, and to invoke a calmer nature. Meditation can help us to alleviate stress and take time for ourselves so that we are not keeping our bodies and our minds in a constant state of panic.

Start by concentrating on one thing—concentrate on your breath, concentrate on the flame of a candle—and you will realize how cluttered the mind is, how much we jump from one thought to the other. Mostly, we find the same thoughts coming up over and over again because, on a daily basis, we think up to ninety-eight percent of the same thoughts as yesterday, and that can be dangerous. As we go deeper and deeper into thoughts and memories, the untruth in them can often become true in our minds through repetition. In meditation, we should focus on clarity.

As our minds are always busy or want to be busy, the use of a mantra within a meditation can be a helpful way of concentrating to calm down the mind. You might start with the sacred word like, "OM," that you repeat in your mind or even with your voice. This occupies the mind and stops it from thinking about daily things like work. When you inhale, you say, "OM," and when you exhale, you say, "OM." If you have no relationship to this mantra in the beginning, just say, "I inhale," when you inhale, and, "I exhale," when you exhale. Do not be surprised if you do this and thoughts are still coming up. That is totally normal. Just observe the process and keep going.

If we have too much yang energy in us, it is obviously very hard to just sit down and meditate. We have to burn off some of this moving energy to get into a quieter place. This is where the asanas, or yoga postures, come into play. The poses in a yoga class can be very physical and strengthening, and may even make you sweat a lot. If you go, for example, to an ashtanga yoga class where you are working out in yang energy (high heart rate, producing heat), you can plan to sweat.

Yoga postures are also needed to prepare the body and mind to be able to sit in meditation. Yoga helps to get rid of tension and contraction in the body. If your body experiences pain in the sitting postures, it is hard to concentrate on breath. Lower back pain or tight hips can keep you away from meditation as you might find it uncomfortable. This is why it is important to find a comfortable seat for meditation or a walking option. Do not force yourself into a yogic crossed legged pose—that is not the need or goal of meditation. Sit on a chair or wherever you feel comfortable.

If just sitting is still too hard for you in the beginning, try a walking meditation, or sit for at least two minutes. A walking meditation can take place in a park, in your garden even, or on the beach—wherever you can walk in silence with your own thoughts, with yourself. While you are walking, simply focus on what you see around you, focus on your breath, feel your inhalations and exhalations, observe your breath, become aware of what is happening in your body through your breath. This process is about becoming aware and getting in contact with yourself.

Another option to help you get into meditation is a CD or DVD. You can also find many guided meditations on the internet. For example, on YouTube, you can search for meditations that guide you through a few minutes. Sit down, listen, and let the video guide you as to how to sit and what to focus on (maybe it is a meditation focusing on breath or your emotions). Just be open and follow through the process. The more often you do it, the easier it will become. It might even become a habit once you feel the difference in your body and mind! You will feel the results of the time you are taking for meditation; the time you are taking for your wellness.

The three most common meditations are the transcendental meditation (TM), mindful meditation (which is based on stillness and calming the mind), and Kundalini meditation, where mantras (word or sound to focus on), breath work (pranayama), mudras (hand positions), and some physical movements are used. If you are a beginner, I recommend starting with the mindful meditation at home or to look for a meditation teacher and try what suits you best.

The main objective of meditation is to calm the mind and to bring you into yin energy, to become quiet and connect with your higher Self.

How to meditate:

1. Take time for meditation. It is easy to say that you do not have time, but you should make it possible, even if it is just for one minute in the beginning.

2. Create a space where you can sit down, become quiet, and maybe light a candle and an incense stick to help bring you into a different state of mind.

3. Sit crossed legged on a yoga mat or cushion or on a chair, with a straight spine, and your hands on your knees. If you use a chair, do not lean back against the back of the chair. Sit with a straight spine because you want to stay fully alert.

4. Close your eyes, connect yourself with your breath, let the breath flow, and follow the breath through your nose and into your lungs, into your rib cage, and then see how it feels when the breath comes out. And again, breathe in. Where do you feel it this time? Is it deeper? Longer? Just observe, follow the breath, and then let it out.

5. If you are more of an emotional person, connect yourself with your heart center, and stay concentrated on your heart.

6. If you are more of an intellectual person, connect yourself with your third eye chakra and stay concentrated on that point.

7. Take a few cycles of breath by just observing where you feel it, stretch the breath longer, and feel how the body and mind become more still.

Do not be frustrated or discouraged if it seems very difficult in the beginning to focus and concentrate on one single thing. This takes time and practice. But with time and practice, you gain power and control over your thoughts, and you might learn to stop them completely. You will learn how to separate yourself from your thoughts. That means that when a thought appears, you can make the decision whether or not it is a valuable thought and if you want to keep it.

When we do not take awareness of our thoughts, we believe in them at surface level, but our true thoughts and beliefs are something much deeper. A belief is a thought you are thinking all the time, over and over again, so you start believing it, and it becomes your truth. For example, if you think all the time, *I am a lazy person*, or, *I am not loved*, you start believing those thoughts and they become your truth. But that truth is just made up by your thoughts through a certain situation you lived. As soon as we become aware of this whole system, you can start to influence your feelings, emotions, and your whole life. In this way, you can get rid of imbalances in your life, especially ones that might namely be products of your thoughts.

In yoga, the mind is compared to a lake, and only when the lake is still, no waves, no currents that whirl the sand of the lake bottom up into the water, can the ground be seen and all is clear. It is the same with the mind. When all is still, you can see what's going on and you can understand more clearly so that you may take the right action and make the best decisions.

By implementing a meditation practice into your life, you start to balance yang energy with yin energy, and you start to become more conscious and aware. By working on your breath in meditation (pranayama techniques), you will see major results in your body and mind. Researchers have shown how meditation affects your health and the brain. Just the addition of oxygen through breathing meditation incites a lot of healthy changes in the body such as improved digestion, clearer thinking, better sleep, which all means feeling more balanced in life. Sometimes, we just need to breathe more deeply to connect and feel more balanced. Meditation is an easy way to bring this into your life.

Chapter 6

When Is Too Much Yang?

Most people today lead a life focused on yang. We don't do it consciously. It is just the energy that is out there. It is in the way our society functions and in what we're taught we have to do to be on the top. The internet, social media, information overflow—all of this takes part in that fast moving energy with which we feel we have to keep up with.

Yin and yang energies are found everywhere in life. If you are a person with a lot of willpower and you are action oriented, you are more yang. In contrast, you are more yin when you know how to relax, you are able to make time for yourself, you practice meditation, and connect with nature. The question is, how can you stay in balance with yin and yang, in your own nature, in your own life, and within the environment you are living in? When we never take a break, calm down, and bring ourselves back to yin energy, the body becomes imbalanced. The body can only take a certain amount of yang energy before it begins to seek out balance.

Within our relationships, we should be checking to see if we are in balance. A more yang person is more sociable and extroverted, reaches out to others, and likes to share. The yin way to relate to others is more introverted—you listen and are thoughtful, perceptive, compassionate, and understanding. It's easier for a yin person to turn inward, receive, and understand others in order to build trust. Yin energy is used in a more sensitive way to relate.

The job and the career you have chosen also gives an indication about your personality. Yang energy chooses jobs that involve hard work or something physically demanding like gardening, cleaning, construction work, heavy lifting, etc. The yin careers are more related to mental work, education, reading, writing, singing, playing instruments, drawing, painting, all kinds of creative work, as well as meditation, teaching, baking and cooking.

Your sleep habits also reflect characteristics of yin and yang. If you have an imbalance in your life, you will certainly see it in your sleeping routine. The evening is the natural time for yin energy to flow through your body, mind, and spirit. Yin promotes rest, relaxation, and good sleep. It helps us to rejuvenate our bodies during the night. Those who are yin deficient will likely have trouble falling and staying asleep, experience recurrent nightmares, and may potentially suffer from insomnia.

If you are feeling tired all day long, even though you had lots of sleep, it may signal a deficiency in yang energy. Our yang energy regenerates itself at night. Yang energy peaks during the day and is strongest at noon. In the evening, yang gently gives way to yin. Without enough yang in the body, you can lose energy, and many individuals find themselves waking up exhausted, regardless of their sleep patterns.

But if your mind is full of stress, anxiety, or emotional conflicts, you cannot find rest and relaxation. Nutrition can also play a role in your yin and yang balance or imbalance. Not only what kind of food you eat, but also what time you eat can cause imbalance. If you eat late at night, it can disrupt your sleep as this affects your metabolism.

Your exercise routine can also affect your balance of the yin and yang modus. In general, exercise promotes good sleep. Vigorous exercise should be done in the morning or late afternoon as this is the time when your body is in yang modus, while a yoga class in the evening promotes yin energy in preparation for sleep.

Finding balance between yin and yang is not always easy. I understand, as I have been there—you feel completely exhausted when you have too much yang, believe me. Of course, we can push our bodies to persevere, but I have learned that you pay a high price for this—with your body, your family, your quality time with friends, on your whole life.

I obviously had too much yang in my life for many years, but couldn't see it. I pursued extremes. I tried a yang approach exemplified through crash diets and many superintense workout systems. My work life and family life became stressful and suffered as a result. My life became one-dimensional and even dangerous. Instead of enjoying my workouts, I tried to work through extreme pain, which is typical yang style—blocking out important signs of distress and increasing the risk for injury. I did what I often see my clients doing—using Ibuprofen or other painkillers to be able to take on more pain.

People who are intensity junkies work to extremes for a certain amount of time. Then, they become so frustrated with pain and exhaustion that they end up on the couch, doing nothing for a few weeks until the next extreme wave hits them and pushes them back to the gym. There is still this opinion that a hard workout is a good workout and only that will lead to results, but no, it won't.

I still wonder today why I lived this way, and why other people still live this way. Is it really what society expects of us? Is it that we just can't see it because we are not aware? Is it that we all have fear of not being good enough? Whatever the reason, and each of us have our own "good" reasons, if you want to change, and especially if you want to improve your quality of life, you have to figure out how to find balance. On a scale of one to ten, where you are in terms of yin or yang? Do you exercise in yin or yang? Do you eat in yin or yang?

I developed the desire to become a fitness coach when I felt the most yang in my life. I wanted to know exactly what to do to gain muscle weight, to build my body, and to go through the pain for major results. But by becoming a fitness coach, I began to understand why this kind of work can become useless and really harmful to the body. Alternatively, I also learned when and how it can help you and improve your health and happiness. As a health and fitness coach, the wellbeing of my clients is the most important thing. We hurt ourselves when we push ourselves too much. The tendency to focus on repetitive, physically punishing methods of exercise at the expense of our own wellbeing may well find its roots in some of our more deeply held Western values.

Going to the gym three times a week for an hour is not the way to change your body, lifestyle, and happiness. No. You must learn to quiet your mind, to tell yourself that you want to do something *for* your body, not *to* it. Changing your life, health, and nutrition can be complex. You can't split the mind from the body, or divide yourself into muscle groups, work them in isolation, and expect to improve performance and health.

I have not seen many people in the gym who really improve their health or lifestyle. Of course, exercising is always good for the body and improves something, but there is much more to it than just lifting weights. It is more mind work, personal development, and lots of psychological work. Some people who are already over stressed and living with too much yang energy might need some "hardcore" exercise to get rid of their excess yang energy. For instance, running can be a form of exercise used to destress, but you also have to understand where the stress comes from, why something is stressing you, and what complementary form of exercise/food/lifestyle you could implement to bring balance to it. If you already have too much yang, you cannot balance it out with more yang. You need to bring in some yin.

I am not judging the fitness world, and of course, for some people, fitness and other yang workouts are exactly what they need at that time. It is obviously also what I needed for many years, but looking back now, yang exercise was not what helped me to improve my health. I used a lot of that to run away from the real problems in my life. I used my workouts to compensate. I am not sure if I should have been able to understand it earlier in my life, but I hope this book helps you to think about what you are doing now and helps you to determine if there might be a better way. Become aware of your needs so that you may find balance.

Chapter 7

The Eastern
Yin Approach

At the other end of the fitness spectrum is the yin approach. It is an internal, holistic, and exploratory approach. Yin practices include things like yoga, Pilates, NIA, tai chi, qigong, Feldenkrais, and some forms of dance and martial arts. All of these practices require full participation of the body, mind, and spirit.

Yin exercises tend to leave you feeling rejuvenated instead of depleted. Meditative walks, easy swims, stretching, and yin yoga are all examples of restorative exercises. Corrective exercise, in the form of rolling and dynamic stretching, all of which focus on improving movement quality rather than targeting muscles with more reps, sets, speed and mileage, can also fall into the yin category.

Each time I did some sort of yin dominated exercise during my highly stressed life phase, I started to feel more connection to myself and to my emotions, and I came to understand, "Ah, that's why I prefer yang exercise—more running, more stressing—because I do not have to feel the real feeling," like the sadness, the hunger for understanding, the need for communication, and the awareness of my Self. But once I made it through a yoga class, I felt the difference. I felt rejuvenated. I finally felt a sense of balance.

When I live more in yin energy (I have to admit, sometimes too much yin), I feel so much more connected with my body while doing Pilates. My body has a healthier structure and posture. I feel immediately taller after a session. The chance of hurting myself is low, and I really feel good and loved after a session. The same goes for yoga, especially after a yin yoga session. I feel so alive and calm at the same time, it is almost hard to explain.

Presence and attention are key aspects to the yin approach, making a yin-style training session not just a workout for your body but also for your brain, your organs, and all of your body tissue and nervous system as well.

The difference from a yang workout is that you forget the end result. In yin, you are not there to count repetitions, rather you are more in the moment. You are connected. You feel your body. You experience your body, moment by moment, and this inspires self-love. Through yin, you are given a fascinating and enjoyable feeling.

Yin style movement also affects the parasympathetic nervous system, dispelling stress and leaving you calm and focused. Simultaneously, these movements improve your coordination, balance, and control. I often see clients who have no bodily control or feeling at all. This is most common in people with sedentary jobs, even those who exercise regularly. But yin-style movement helps restore connection and experience with one's own body.

Our bodies would greatly benefit from just walking fifteen minutes a day, but many people find it difficult to detach from work and get moving. There are so many easy ways we can bring movement into our daily lives so that we may improve our health and reduce stress levels.

I am always happy to see that where I live, people still walk, jog, or go to the ocean to do regular exercises. My favorite picture is of an old woman, around seventy years old, walking through the little village from her house to the beach in her swim suit, equipped only with a towel, and of course, no mobile phone. Many of the older people here know about and appreciate the healthy benefits of the ocean and its salt water. The ocean is therapeutic in so many ways as it is rich in minerals and microelements, which help to detoxify the body, soothe the skin, and calm the mind.

Younger people think that by running at the gym and lifting weights they will be healthy and become fit, but most of them are just bringing more stress and yang energy into their lives. Sometimes, I see clients who answer the phone while running on the treadmill. I can understand if you are a doctor on call, but otherwise, this does not make sense at all. When you are distracted, you totally miss the point of what you are doing. And after a session in the gym like this, still stressed, they rush back to work while eating a sandwich in the car. Sorry, but that is not healthy. We must find out what it is we need to find balance for better health and for recreation.

Improving your fitness results can be much easier than you think. Find something that you like, and I mean really like, which does not feel like a punishment or another task that needs to be done. The intensity of your workout should be moderate, at a level which challenges your body, but does not harm you by using too much weight or by pushing you through a long run. You should slow down once in a while, and learn how to breathe deeply and mindfully, learn how to move with grace. There is no need to rush through an exercise. It will probably hurt and be less likely to yield a result. With Pilates, I have learned how important it is to work efficiently so that the result is positive. There is no need to rush or push more weight or volume. Doing so will just increase your chance of injury.

The secret to less injuries is in how you do your exercises. Correct form is very important. I see it in class when people are pushing or rushing through push-ups, speeding through crunches with a crazy and unhealthy body posture. This is the best predictor of injury. We need to always be aware of the quality of our movements.

So think about yourself for a moment. How would you describe your level of exercise? What motivates you? Do you think you are doing enough or too much? Are you doing the right form of exercise? Listen deep in your heart. Maybe you've known for a long time that you wish to do something else, but you just didn't know that there was another way; that maybe a ten-minute walk a day could help you more than the hour run you're taking on the weekends. Just analyze without judging your feelings or thoughts. Start by being honest and figure out what else is out there, and what feels right for you.

Chapter 8

Finding the Right Balance For You

Though most exercises draw on either the intensity of yang energy or the calm and focus of yin, as always, the most successful exercise programs draw elements from both. Using a more balanced approach, yin and yang complement and build on one another. The physical skill, control, and mindfulness developed through yin training is enhanced by the force and power of yang training, and vice versa.

One way of doing this is to simply include attitudes from both schools in your exercise program. To build up your fitness, short and intense workouts (like interval training) are the most effective and time efficient way to do so.

Including yoga or another restorative-type class once or twice a week, plus some kind of soft tissue bodywork once or twice a month, is necessary to find balance for your body and mind. Unfortunately, I see many people who push themselves through hard workouts to gain strength, but they never get enough stretching in. A body can endure this for some time, maybe even for some years, but this kind of training often results in a lot of pain, muscle and ligament trauma, and worn down joints. If you want to stay healthy and balanced while having fun, treat yourself like a world class champion. Exercise like one, eat like one, and love yourself and your body.

Today, I love to sit down for meditation to help me feel restored. I understand how powerful that technique is and what it can do for my body, my health, and my happiness. The changes I've made through meditation are innumerable and I could never go back to the person I was before. Meditation is the most powerful practice in helping you to understand yourself, your body, your mind, your beliefs, life, and to how to heal your soul.

While meditation can be spiritual, becoming more spiritual does not mean you become religious. You simply become aware of what you are doing, of what happened to you, what you do to others, and you come to deeply understand your desires, values, life story, and your ability to change whatever you want to change. Spirituality and meditation helps you to overcome your narrow and ego-driven way of life (well, it might take a whole lifetime to do that), and expands your understanding for a more fulfilled experience.

"Meditation means the mind is turned back upon itself.
The mind stops all the thought waves and the world stops.
Your consciousness expands. Every time you meditate,
you will keep your growth."

-Swami Vivekananda

In the yin and yang symbol, we see two parts—black and white, masculine and feminine, hard and soft, sun and moon—but there's a little dot of the dark in the light, and a little of the light in the dark. This is to show that every good yin practice has a little yang in it, and vice-versa. Yin and yang is a symbiotic relationship, there is an interdependency, moving and swirling together and becoming one another. It's a process of continual transformation and finding balance.

Maybe you just need to start to shift your approach or your perspective on the things that you are doing, and you might quickly feel more balance. For example, if you take yoga but you feel like you need more exercise, you can attend a more demanding class, one that is more advanced with more yang. You do not necessarily need to put in an extra hour of running or weight lifting. You can find what you need in yoga through meditation and breathing.

Sometimes we think it is too complicated to incorporate more exercise into our lives because we sit for too many hours at a desk. You do not have to sign up for a gym that puts pressure on you. What about a regular walk on the weekends or evenings in your neighborhood? If you have the chance, like me, to be close to the ocean, you can walk or run there, jump in the ocean, or swim. Thirty-minutes is enough, and while you are there, or anywhere else in nature, remember to just sit down on a wooden log, appreciate nature, and breathe. By doing this, you bring more yin into your life and into your workouts by simply paying attention to your surroundings. Nature is also very healing. Allow the energy of the forest, the ocean, the birds to enter your mind. Be aware and it will shift your perceptions and perspective of life.

No matter what you choose for activity, the way you do it is more important than what you do. Even a classical yin yoga class can challenge your body, a tai chi class may become infused with force and intensity, or even the weightlifting you are doing can be meditative if you do it with awareness and not while staring at a TV. It is also important that you like and enjoy what you are doing, and that you are able to be present for every moment of it!

My approach to sports, exercise, and fitness has totally changed over the last twenty years. I used to be like everybody else—the more the better; the more pain, the more effective; the more I push myself, the more I will be accepted (by myself and others), and the more value I will have. Wrong! But that was also exactly what I did in my life as an engineer. I was in this group consciousness and wanted to stay on top, faster, higher, better, which meant I abandoned myself, my body, and my mind.

With time, I realized that I mostly did lots of stretching because that was the part I really liked. Stretching is where I finally felt relaxed in my muscles. I felt like I'd traveled in my spirit to a different place, and that is exactly what, I thought, our society needs more of.

When I started fitness coaching and working in the gym, I realized that what people really need, the people who are looking for balance, not the professional athletes, is to feel good in their body. They need to know what to eat and how to eat right, and how to get out of the treadmill of life, which pushes us to reach for unrealistic goals. Our society is fueled by pressure, competition, and pace! It hurts me to watch clients who are totally unable to run five minutes on a treadmill, but who want to push through ten minutes or pile on weights, as if they have to show me how "good" they are. With so much tension and pressure in life, why should we put more tension and pressure on ourselves in the form of stress through weights on our bodies?

WE NEED TO WAKE UP,

UNDERSTAND OUR REAL DESIRES,

AND FINALLY START LOVING OURSELVES!

Chapter 9

Finding Balance With Food

In traditional Chinese medicine, every food has an energy, and the food you eat gives energy to your body. Yin food is more cooling and often raw (expanding), whereas yang food is hot and spicy (contracting). The hot climate is yang and the cold winter time is yin. Now, you probably understand that we crave more hot and spicy yang food in winter to be in balance with the yin season, and that it is easier to eat raw food in the summer when the season is yang. So, by nature, we are designed to find balance, and the more you are connected with your body, the more you understand what you need.

When we don't find balance naturally or consciously, the body will find it on its own and become reactive. For example, a heart attack can be seen as a way for your body to find balance; to put you on rest; to give you a break. The body can only take a certain amount of stress, and if we do not understand or do not listen to our body's warning signs, nature will find its own way.

Food plays an important role in our health and balance. That's why it is so important to take a look at the way you nurture your body and mind and if there is room for improvement to get rid of imbalances. An easy tool you can use to understand your connection to food is a food-mood journal. Here, you take awareness and write down everything that you eat while observing your body's reactions, your mood, your level of tiredness, etc.

FOOD-MOOD JOURNAL

You should not start changing anything in your diet. Simply spend the next few days being conscious of what you eat, when you eat, why you eat (are you really hungry?), and how you feel before and after eating. Write it all down—everything, even if you have a piece of chewing gum. By keeping a food-mood journal, you will start to get an idea of what side of the scale you are on: Do you eat more yin or yang food? Do you feel cold often? Do you crave hot/warm food or more cool/raw food? Which food gives you an energy boost, and which tears you down or fatigues you? Is there food that makes you angry or moody? Just be aware.

1. List the food you ate and the time you ate it

2. My hunger level was: 0-10

3. Before I ate, I felt hungry/bored/moody/happy

4. After I ate, I felt hungry/bored/moody/happy

5. My energy level before eating was: 0-10

6. My energy after eating was: 0-10

OBSERVATIONS

- I always feel _____ when I eat _____.

- After raw food, I feel _____.

- Eating dairy makes me _____.

- My energy level was 0-10, but now it's 0-10.

As you go on testing which food is doing what to your body, only crowd out one food group at a time. For example, leave dairy out for ten days, then implement it back in. Then, take gluten out for ten days, then implement it back in. Of course, it takes a while (weeks to months), but you can be sure that you will get a lot of information about your body, how your body functions, your metabolism, and your digestion.

Once you've got a pretty good picture of your eating habits and their effects on your body and mind, you can start playing around with your food. Leave some sort of food out—maybe go ten days without dairy, and again, be aware of how your mood might be different or if your body feels different. Continue keeping your food-mood journal to really understand your body and mind in connection with food and your habits around food. You might find that you always eat sweets when you feel stressed or tired, or that you binge on something because you just feel bored. There might be a high chance that you understand that you eat even if you are not hungry, but just to be occupied or distracted from an emotion.

If you already have a daily yoga practice in your life, you might feel a difference in your asanas when you change your food habits. You might become more flexible or more focused.

After you have taken a food group out of your diet for ten days, implement it back into your meal plan. Your body will react if there is a problem.

As soon as you become more aware of your food-mood connection, you can better understand what your body needs in different seasons. In the winter time, we usually need more hot/warm food like soups and steamed vegetables. In the summer, it is easier to sustain with raw food, salads, and fruits. We often are less hungry in the summer, but need more water.

Because of your unique genetics, the environment you live in, your blood type, and your body's specific demand for nutrients and calories (Are you moving a lot or sitting all day in front of a computer?), everyone is different and has different needs. This is the definition of bio-individuality. It is also the reason that no one diet can work for everybody in the same way. Learn to listen to your body and to find your unique needs.

Like they say: You are what you eat!

YIN RELAXING

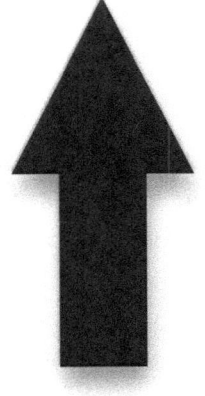

medication/drugs
alcohol/caffeine
sugar
dairy: milk/cream/yogurt
oil
white flour
fruit/nuts
leafy green vegetables
sea vegetables

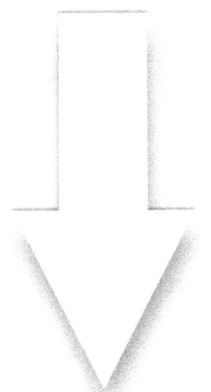

root vegetables, grains
beans
fish
chicken
hard cheese
red meat
miso and tamari
eggs
salt

YANG CONTRACTING

(Figure 1)

In figure 1, you see a schema of the yin and yang concept regarding food. Do not get me wrong, as the title of the book says, yin is the new black. I do not want to tell you to go just for yin food now. For the majority of the population, yang food is found in higher percentages on our plates (the more processed the food, the more yang properties) than yin food. For many, eggs, meat, and cheese is eaten in bigger portions than anything else.

However, if you have too much yang food, your body is contracting muscles, gets stiff, migraines and headaches might appear more often, high blood pressure can result from being out of balance, sleeplessness, digestive problems, and contracted muscles can pull on joints, causing you back pain. The reason for this is obvious. Yang is often salty, processed food and high in sodium, which contracts muscles and cells. That's why you feel an imbalance. When you are out of balance, your body will show you through illness, pain, and bad moods. Instead of reaching for a quick and short term solution, it is important to find balancing long-term solutions for your health and happiness.

Again, finding balance on your plate is the goal. Figure 1 shows a very simple module—if you stay around the middle line, you should find balance with root vegetables, beans, grains, green vegetables, and fruits.

Keep in mind that our bodies are also made through the food we eat. Our cells reproduce themselves over our lifetime with the nutrients you feed your body. Food is fuel for your body and mind. When your cells replace or renew, they will be made out of the food that you have put into your body, so how you nurture yourself is important for your cells.

The energy in your food depends on where the food comes from, the energy properties in the area where the food was grown and harvested. By understanding the energies around your meals, you can make the right choices to get the energy you are seeking for your life. Food is not just nutrients, vitamins, and minerals, it is energy.

Vegetables have lighter energy than proteins. The meat from a tortured animal has, of course, a different energy than meat sourced from a more peaceful existence. If you look back to the chart of yin and yang food, you can see that if you eat mostly yang food, it will put your body in yang energy—your body and your energy will be contracting and stressed. As nature is looking for balance, while eating lots of yang food, your body will attract yin food in order to feel relaxed. For example, with a heavy meal of meat and eggs, you may crave alcohol and sugar to help you balance. This is why people crave a glass of wine or a beer after a long, hard day at work, as it is just natural that your body is looking for something relaxing after a stressed day in the office. Now you might say, "Well, that's great if I'm just finding my balance when I need a glass of alcohol!" You can guess, though, that it is not like this. A better way would be to eat a more balanced diet to begin with.

The body also needs different energy to digest different kinds of food. Often, cooked meals take a lot of energy from our body to digest and metabolize, whereas raw food gives us energy. But for some people, raw food can be more difficult to digest, so it is always worth looking at your individual capacities and needs. Becoming aware of how your body feels when you eat is the first step to understanding your way to find balance.

In yoga philosophy and Ayurveda, it is said that raw food has more "prana," which is life force energy from the Universe. So if you eat life force, you get life force.

As you see, food is a major factor that contributes to balance or imbalance. Signs of imbalance related to food include:

- sleeping problems, insomnia

- anxiety, fear, depression

- headaches, migraines

- bloat, constipation

- digestive problems

- food cravings

- inability to lose weight

- irritable bowel syndrome (IBS)

- skin problems

- libido problems

- chronic fatigue syndrome

- silent inflammation

By finding out which food is good or bad for you, you get the chance to get rid of imbalances like digestion and sleep problems. Otherwise, these imbalances can lead to more stress and more imbalances in your life.

Chapter 10

Finding Balance with Yin Yoga Flow and Breathing

Before I came to yin yoga, I was a strong advocate for hatha yoga, power yoga, and other kinds of very active classes. As I said, I took hours of spinning classes, ran marathons, went biking—everything to avoid thinking about and feeling what was going on in my life. Me, sitting down to relax? No way. But in the last several years of my healing practice, I've come to understand, for myself and for my clients, that we have to calm down. We have to get into ourselves, connect to our bodies and our minds to understand what is going on in our tissues (the issue in the tissue), to understand why we are unhappy and unhealthy.

Yin is seen as the darkness, the night, and yang as the light and the sun. Both sides are complementing each other and necessary in nature. Through yoga, we can find balance in our bodies and minds. Here, I would like to show you how to use yin yoga to get rid of imbalances in your life so that you can feel more happiness and joy.

Personally, when I started with yin yoga, I had the feeling that, with yin, I was touching my dark side. Being for four, five, or even six minutes in the same pose brings you to places in your mind and body where you usually never go. As long as we are moving our bodies or are occupied, we are kind of disconnected from ourselves. But being still, in body and mind, makes you observe yourself, what you think and feel. You have to face it. You cannot escape.

When I completed my certificate course in yin yoga with Ishta yoga in NYC through Yogiraj, Ulrica Norberg, I was ready to embrace a lot of darkness and face a lot of bad stuff I knew was still in me. I felt ready to go to this teacher training, not only to become certified, but because I was sure it would change my life. I had done a lot of healing already, but I knew there was still "stuff" sitting somewhere in my body that I was holding onto that wasn't serving me. The opposite was the case. It was holding me from being free, from doing things I wished I could do, but was still afraid of.

When I laid down every day for ten days in a row, sometimes for two yin sessions a day, I have to admit, I cried a lot. Thoughts like, "I do not want to suffer anymore," suddenly appeared, and then I thought of all the suffering in my life; those days that were pretty dark. I did not know how to continue—thoughts of ending my life when I was a kid, crying after a breakup, bad moods because I didn't know what I wanted, everything came up again and everything wanted a voice.

When this "stuff" is coming up, it often starts with giggling, then turns into laughter, which transforms into cries. And yes, that is the moment where you have to open up and just let go. What we usually do in situations like this is avoid the feeling and compensate with moving, running away, or eating something in order to not feeling it anymore, and just push it down. But no, this is the time to face it, accept it, respect it, even honor it, and then let it go.

Anger comes out a lot, mostly in hip opener poses, and I have never met a student who was not facing this dark emotion in some capacity. Grief is another suppressed friend that often shows up. When I teach, I can often see it in people's faces. You can literally see the pain and the sadness looking for a pathway to come out. The connective tissues hold it back for many years, nicely covered under very tight muscles or even scar tissue, but suddenly, it is there. Even by stretching your hamstrings for a few minutes, your body folds up and brings all the stories back that you were carrying around. In hip openers, we especially touch the liver meridian, and the liver is the organ which stores anger, so when stretching and teasing it, anger comes up, as if it was just waiting for this moment.

When I do healing sessions on clients and acknowledge what a body has to bear in a lifetime, I sometimes wonder why we are not sicker than we are. A body can really take a lot on, but on the other hand, when it has had enough, it knows. I prefer to take control and change consciously, to decide and understand what is hindering or blocking me, and to work on it. Otherwise, finding myself in a situation where my anger comes up uncontrolled and jumps into other people's faces doesn't help me to heal.

We carry all situations, bad or good, as cellular memory in our bodies. The bad stories, of course, bring pain and suffering, anger, sadness, and the Universe wants us to heal. Either healing will take place in situations where it is not really appropriate (when your boss is triggering you and you just explode, it means something wants to come up), or a disease will be created by all the negative emotions you are carrying around. So, why not just choose the option to heal actively, consciously, and balance your body through yin yoga?

Yin yoga is a very therapeutic method to get rid of imbalance, and you control it! The fact that you made the decision to take a yin class means you are aware what is going on and that you want to give your body and mind the chance to change and heal in a safe and protected way.

When I saw how many clients ask for a yin session, I understood that this is our deepest wish—to heal and to feel good. It wasn't just me who'd had enough of suffering. I guess the time is right for everybody as the stress, the information overflow, the fast food, and yang influence in our lives is too high and we are looking for balance and peace inside.

Another funny thing that appeared during my certification class is that after each pose on my left side, I had to get up out of class to the bathroom. At the time, I could not figure out why! But I had stored so much stuff in my bladder, which obviously needed to get out, and I am very happy to have let it go. It makes so much sense to me now, as I had suffered my whole life with bladder and kidney infections. No wonder these organs needed some healing and love! The work on our organs through a yin class is amazing. Organs are yin parts of the body, just like the tissues, the ligaments, and the joints are. So everything that is stored in these body parts gets touched and activated. You see the results immediately, and even by looking in the mirror in the evening, it was so visible that something had changed. Within the ten-day course, my skin had completely cleared up and my puffy eyes (kidney imbalance) were gone for good as well.

So let's have a quick look again at how yin yoga helps to get rid of imbalances in your body and even in your life:

- A yin yoga session quiets the mind.

- Yin yoga balances the body and mind through breathing techniques.

- Yin yoga stretches the connective tissue, which is like a net in your body and connects everything (head to toe)!

- A yin pose works so deep in the body that it acts on meridians, which we know from traditional Chinese medicine and acupuncture, works on the organs (especially kidney, bladder, gall bladder, liver, stomach, lungs).

- Yin yoga promotes increased blood flow and circulation in organs, tissue, and joints.

- Yin yoga improves your sleep.

- Yin yoga increases your energy level.

- Yin yoga improves your metabolism.

- Yin yoga can completely relax your muscles.

I will offer you a special breathing technique to use with the yin poses. It is a kriya technique called Arowan Awarohan:

*"Offering the inhaling breath into the exhaling breath,
and offering the exhaling breath into the inhaling breath,
the yogi neutralizes both breaths; thus, he releases prana
from the heart and brings life force under his control."*

—The Bhagavad Gita, IV:29

I learned this technique, Arowan Awarohan, at Ishta) yoga in the yoga teacher training. Ulrica Norberg from Sweden, international yoga teacher, writer and Yogiraj at Ishta, connected this breathing technique of Arowan Awarohan with yin yoga poses as it reinforces the relaxation even more. As long as you can breathe comfortably, you are okay.

Arowan Awarohan works on two energetic pathways in the body—

the ascending one, arowan, and the descending one, awarohan. The passageway of these energy lines creates a figure eight in your body on which the breath flows.

Inhalation starts in the pelvis, comes up over the belly, lifts the chest up, goes through the throat, back to the head, up on the back side of the head, and enters the top through bindu, into the middle of the head, ajna chakra. From there, the exhalation goes down through the head, back to C7 (cervical spine), and down through the spine, back into the pelvis, where the next inhalation can start.

You want to feel a regular, smooth breath during this figure eight through your body. After a while, you will feel how the front (rajas) and the back (tamas) of your body comes into balance and you will feel calm and steady (sattvic).

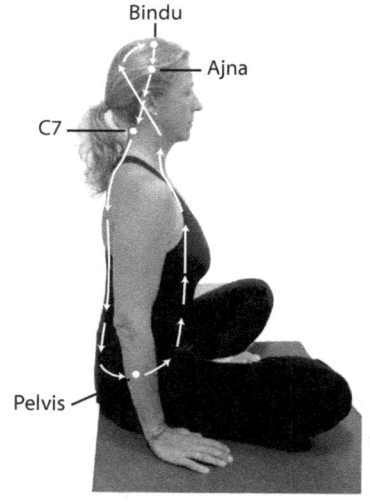

Another advantage of this breathing technique is the awareness of pure consciousness as the central channel in the spinal cord (brahma nadi) is activated.

For me, personally, the advantage of the combination of Arowan Awarohan and the yin poses is a complete observation inside the body and mind. The breathing technique, pratyahara, or the withdrawal of the senses, is the fifth element among the eight stages of Patanjali's Ashtanga yoga, as mentioned in his classical work, *The Yoga Sutras of Patanjali Composed in the 2nd Century BCE*. Combined with the poses, it deepens your observation inside—you can go deeper into it, getting in touch with feelings and emotions.

Though breathing, the inhalation and exhalation, is something natural and happens automatically, we are often out of balance in our breathing. If our breath is short and superficial, it messes with our whole system. For example, metabolism depends on oxygen. Oxygen is needed to nurture our cells and organs and is the most important thing to the brain and nervous system. Mental performance can be improved through extra oxygen supply to the brain, and slower and deeper breathing reduces stress levels. So, keep in mind that food and oxygen are primary nutrition needed to grow, repair, and maintain all body cells and tissues.

Your muscles need oxygen to relax, so for your yin yoga flow, always be aware and breathe slowly and deeply while in a pose. If you can't, change to a more comfortable position so that you can comfortably provide oxygen for your relaxation process.

Even if you cannot find a lot of time to implement the yin yoga flow in your life, figure out how to make time for ten to fifteen minutes of breathing exercises every day. These few minutes a day will make an immediate difference. Add just one or two yin poses with breathing after a long stressed day and you will feel balanced, getting your power and energy back for a healthy life. By starting small, you can at least establish a routine to build upon.

As you don't need to warm up your muscles for these poses, it is easy to get started, get onto the mat and into a pose. The yin pose applies moderate stress to the connective tissues of the body, the tendons, fascia, and ligaments. Herewith it increases the circulation in the joints and improves flexibility. The flow of the subtle energy, "qi," that runs down the meridians in Chinese medicine will also increase. Improved qi flow improves organ health, immunity, and emotional wellbeing.

YIN POSES

The following is an outline of yin poses that I have chosen to give you an overview. However there are many more that you can find, for example with BKS Iyengar in his book 'Light on Yoga'. With these poses here you can begin to build your own flow.

Before you start doing and practicing the yin yoga poses, I recommend that you read through the catalog of poses (asanas), which are in alphabetical order. This gives you an overview. After the catalog of poses, you will find two examples of yin flows. When you feel comfortable, you can pick poses from this collection to create your own flow. Yin poses are usually held for three to five or even six minutes to reach the fascia and the meridians. Always be gentle and aware with your body. I also strongly recommend finding a yoga teacher to take some classes.

ANAHATASANA

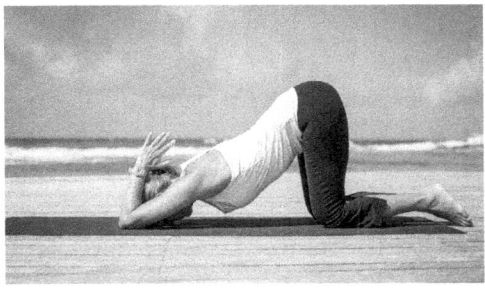

Pose: Keep your hip right above the knees, bottom bones pointing up and back, no compression behind the lumber spine while pressing the elbows into the floor, elbows are shoulder width apart, bring the heart down to the mat and breathe into that area. Feel the opening.

Target area/region: Upper and middle back, heart opening, diaphragm, erector spine, shoulder girdle, trapezius

Options:

- Knees on a towel or blanket, if painful
- Only one arm forward and head resting on the other arm
- Bolster under elbows

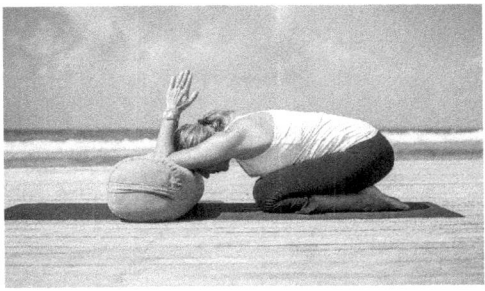

Contraindications:

- Be careful with neck injuries, as it could strain further, so keep your neck long.

- If pain behind shoulder blades appears, use less pressure with arms or widen elbows, and avoid tingling in hands. Otherwise, use Child's Pose.

- If pain behind lumbar spine appears, go into Child's Pose.

ANKLE STRETCH

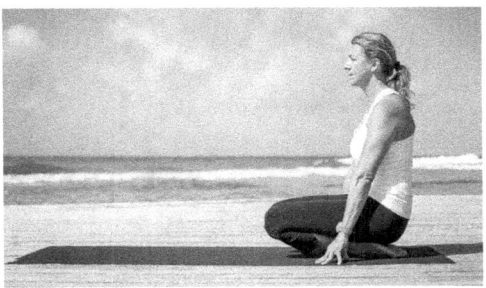

Pose: Sit on your shinbone and keep your feet flat on the mat while sitting on your heels. If you do not feel comfortable here, try with a blanket under the knees. Bring your knees slightly off the mat while having hands on the floor, without falling back with your torso.

Target area: Front of the foot and ankle, deep stretch

Contraindications:

- If you have too much pain in the knee, use a blanket or rolled up towel behind the knees.

- If you have pain in the ankle, try with towel under feet.

- Always respect your body. Remember, maybe the stretch is not for you.

BANANASANA

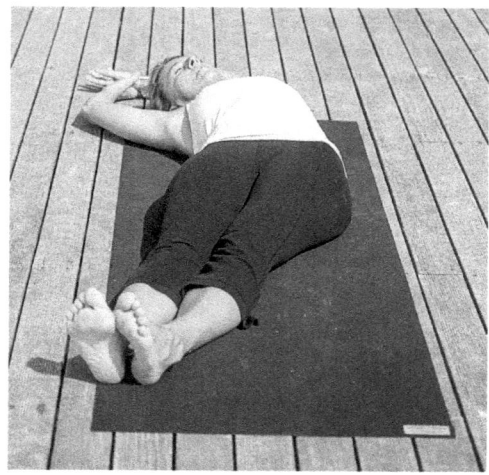

Pose: Lay on your back, legs together, bring both legs to one side and bring arms overhead as well to the same side as feet, keeping shoulder blades down, hips down. When legs and arms are on the right side, grab your left wrist with right hand to get a little pull to the side. On the other side, change wrist. Feel that your body is forming a banana shape. To get out, come back to center, release, and hug your knees for a moment.

Target area/region: Stretch of the side of the body, lateral flexion/obliques, intercostals, iliotibial band

Contraindications:

• You do not want to feel tingling in arms or hands. When your shoulder is coming up on one side, do not stretch too much.

• With lower back pain, do not stretch too far to one side.

BUTTERFLY / HALF BUTTERFLY

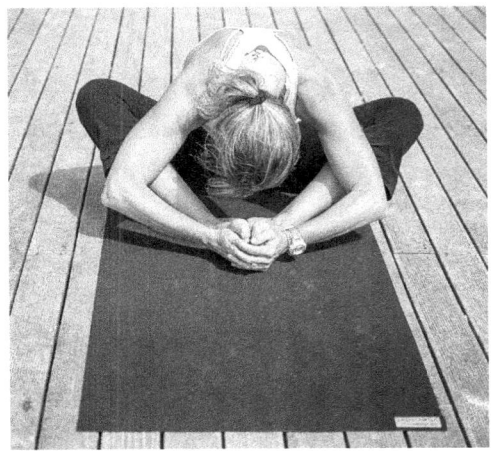

Pose: In most cases, it is recommended to sit on a blanket to have hips higher up, bring knees outside and down, and have your feet touching in front of you. Push your feet a bit forward to form a nice diamond shape with your legs, round the spine, and come down with your head (crown) to your feet.

For the half butterfly, one leg stays straight in front of you and the other one is flexed, foot against the inner thigh.

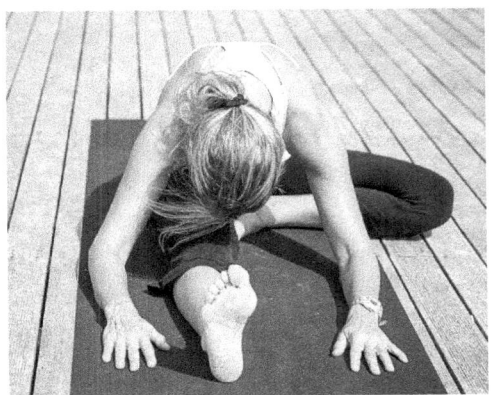

Target region: Lower back muscles, hamstrings (when feet are further away from groin), adductor (when feet are closer to the groin)

Contraindications:

- With sciatica problems, bring hips higher on a cushion, or bolster to have the knees lower than the hip/groin.

- If hip is rolling backward when chest is coming forward, stop, as hip should rotate forward.

- In case of neck problems, use a bolster to rest your head on. Do not pull the head forward (especially with neck problems or injuries like whiplash).

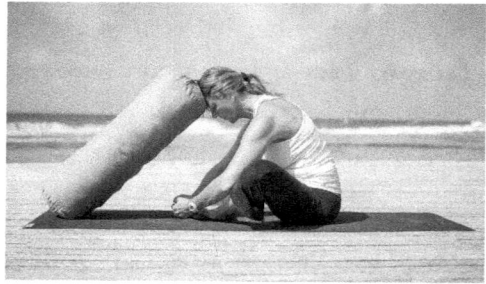

- Avoid flexion of the lower spine. If you have injuries in this area, recline.

- Avoid pulling head down to the feet.

CAMEL

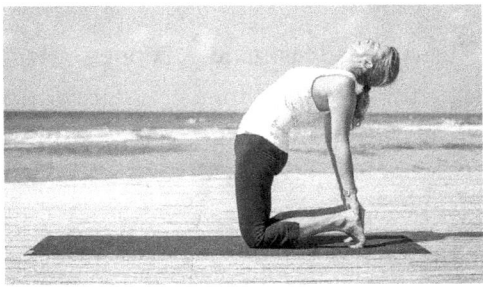

Pose: Keep knees hip distance apart, feet behind line of knees, either on toes (heals are higher up) or feet down on the mat. Open the thighs and the chest to reach one arm after another behind you on the heels.

Target area/region: Opens thighs, arches lumbar spine, opens ankles, stretches hip flexor and opens shoulder and pectoral muscles

Options:

- Just stay on your knees and bring hand on hips or behind lumbar region to open chest with shoulder blades back and down and look up.

- If you are very flexible in the back with no injuries, bring hands behind you on the floor instead of on heels.

- If you have no injuries in the back, you can have your head further back and down.

Contraindications:

- Do not do the pose with spinal injuries, neck injuries, a weak back, or a weak lumbar spine.

- Avoid pinching in lumbar spine.

- Protect your neck while keeping chin toward the chest.

Meridians: Urinary bladder and kidney meridians through compression in sacrum area and lumbar spine, stomach and spleen meridians in thighs, heart and lung meridians through arms, with neck in the back thyroid stimulation

CAT PULLING ITS TAIL

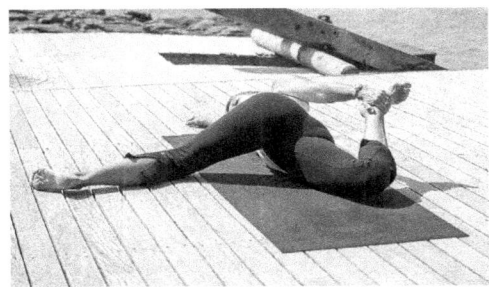

Pose: This pose is an alternative when dragon is too much for your thighs. It is also a little bend in the lumbar region. Lay on your belly and roll a bit on the right side by pulling your left knee up and have the head rested on your right arm. The right leg is straight in the beginning, then you bend the right knee and bring the heel toward the buttocks, reaching back with your left arm to grab the ankle (left hand to right ankle). Pulling softly on your right ankle, to stretch the right thigh and slight compression behind the lower back.

For the other side, you roll again on the belly, pulling the right knee to the right side, left leg is straight, then bend the left knee and roll more on the left side of your body, head is resting on left arm. With right hand, reach for your left ankle and pull gently to get the stretch in your left thigh. To end the pose slowly, let the bent leg go down. Come out of the pose by lengthening both legs still prone and roll on your back.

Target region: Lumbar and sacrum, quadriceps

Options :

- Try laying on a bolster if it is more comfortable.

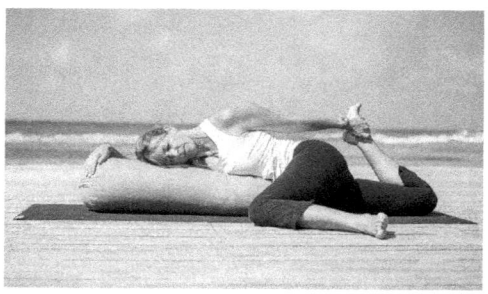

Contraindications:

- With lower back problems, be careful not to arch the back too much.

Meridians: Urinary bladder and kidney meridians when back is arched; stomach and spleen meridian if top of the thigh is activated; with the twist through the side of rib cage, gallbladder is stimulated

CATERPILLAR

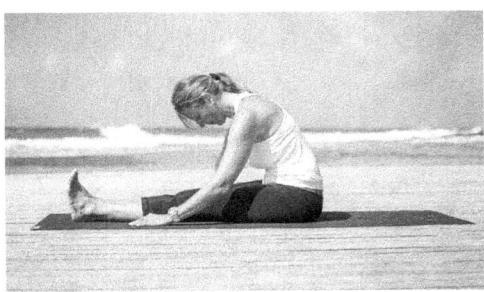

Pose: Sitting with long legs and a straight spine, maybe on a small cushion or blanket, make sure the pelvis is tilted forward. Slowly round the spine and fold forward, let gravity help you, just surrender with arms and shoulders relaxed next to your legs. Make sure legs are relaxed all the time with no contraction in quadriceps. To come out of the pose, slowly roll the spine and neck up.

Target region: Ligaments along back of spine; hamstrings, organs for digestion

Option:

- If the hamstrings are very tight and folding forward is difficult, bend your knees and use a small bolster behind the knees.

- If you are very flexible in your legs, widen legs and come further forward down to mat.

Contraindication:

- In case of neck pain, rest the head on a bolster which is standing up. Or hold head with elbows resting on thighs or on bolster.

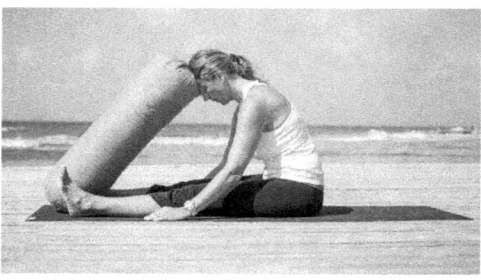

Meridians: Urinary bladder

CHILD'S POSE
The resting pose for all situations.

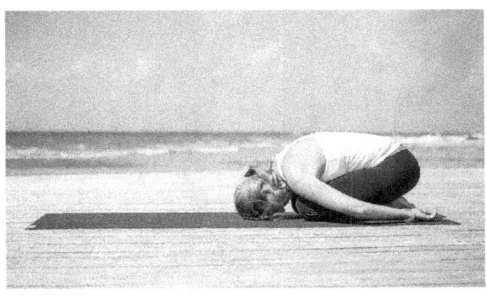

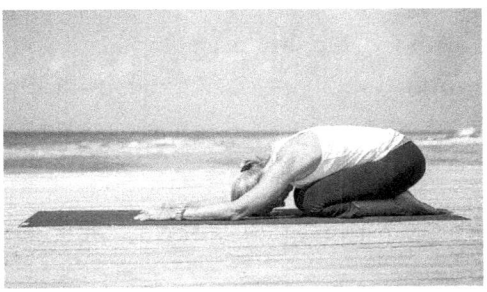

Pose: Start by sitting on your heels and round the spine forward. The forehead should rest on the floor. If head is not touching, use a bolster/blanket under forehead. Close your eyes to relax fully.

Target region: Organs of digestive system, spine

Option:

- When pregnant, open knees to the side and use a bolster.

Contraindication:

- Not recommended if having diarrhea

DANGLING

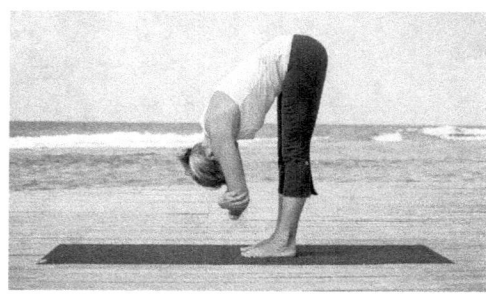

Pose: Stand up with feet hip distance apart, bend your knees slightly to fold forward over the thighs, clasp hands with the opposite side, let gravity hang you down. To get down, always slowly roll the spine "down" or go down in squat.).

Target region: Hamstrings, diaphragm, internal organs, and abdominal muscles

Options:

- Bend knees and keep spine long.

- Sitting in Caterpillar is similar, see if that is an option for you (see contraindication).

- Having the wrist behind legs is an option if you are very flexible.

Contraindications:

- With high blood pressure, glaucoma, or diabetes (sometimes connected with high blood pressure), avoid this pose.

- Roll up slowly to come out of the pose if you have low blood pressure to avoid dizziness, or sit down in a squat to get out of the pose instead of coming up.

- With injuries in lower back, keep spine straight, do not round into flexion of the spine.

Meridians: Urinary bladder, stomach and spleen, meridians in thighs, heart and lung meridians through arms, with neck in the back thyroid stimulation

DRAGON

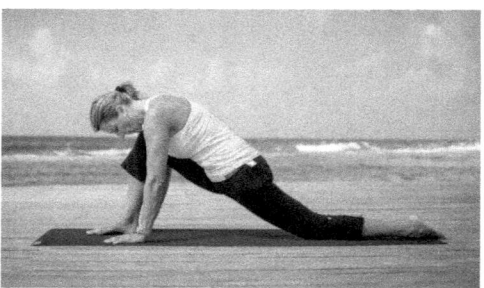

Pose: Start in Down Dog or on knees and step one foot forward in between hands. Make sure knee is above the ankle or a bit further forward. Come down with the back leg to the floor, in order to open in the hip and groin. To open more in the hip, press with back foot into the floor.

Come out of the pose, press your hands into the mat, and swing either the front leg back or come back into Down Dog.

Target region: Hip flexors and quadriceps of back leg (can help with sciatica), ankle, lower back with position of hands up on knee

Options:

- To avoid pain in the knee, maybe a blanket is needed under back of knee.

- Lean against bolster with the back leg (front of quadriceps) and rest against it.

- Bring hands on the front knee, open the chest. This increases the weight over the hip.

- Bring only one hand on the front knee and push the knee out to the side, so the chest rotates to the sky.

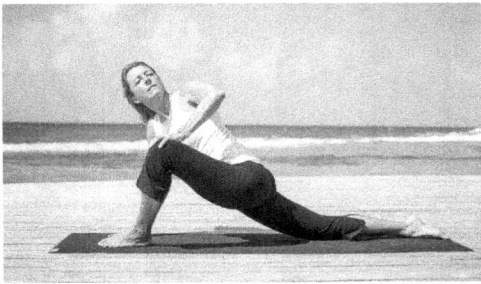

- To go deeper into the pose, come down with your elbows, keep forearms parallel, and press hands into the mat. Forearms can also rest on a bolster.

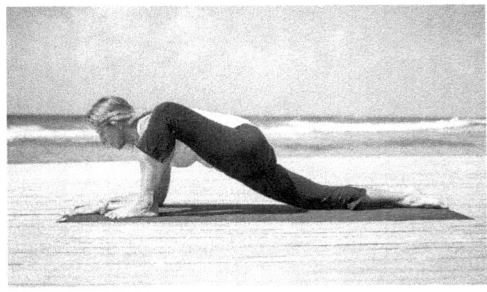

Contraindications:

- If uncomfortable for back of knee (knee cap) or ankle, keep knee up.

- With stiffness in quadriceps and hips of the back leg, the back thigh will stay in 90 degrees to front thigh, then a blanket or cushion under the knee cap recommended to keep the knee cap off the floor.

Meridians: Urinary bladder, stomach and spleen meridians, kidney and gallbladder

DRAGONFLY

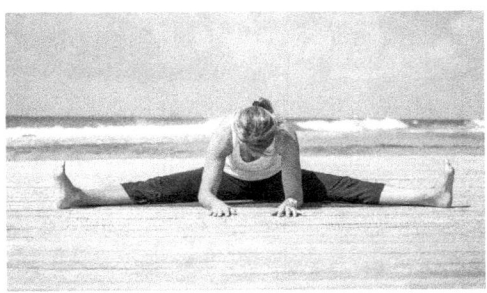

Pose: Start in seated position with legs in front of you, probably a little blanket under your seat will help to bring hips a bit higher and to have a forward tilt in the pelvis. Spread your legs out to the side, with your hands behind the back, can push/slide your hips and legs a bit further forward to widen legs more. Bring hands forward and slowly walk forward to get a nice round spine, do not fall forward. Come slowly up with the spine to get out of the pose. Take time to erect the spine and as well to bring legs closer to the center again. Lean back on your hands to open groin, shake out the legs a bit.

Target region: Inner thighs, back of thighs, hip flexor (groins)

Options:

- To avoid pain in the knee, maybe a blanket is needed under back of knee.

- Lean against bolster with the forehead to support the spine.

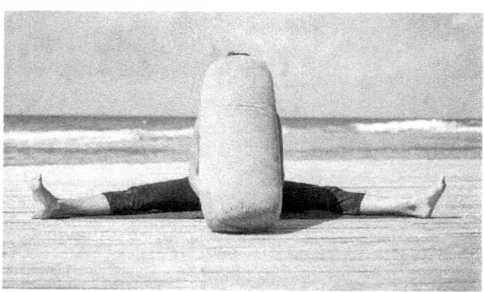

- Sit against the wall with the spine to make sure that pelvis is tilted forward (or use blankets under hips to sit a bit higher up).

Contraindications:

- If uncomfortable for back of knee (knee cap) or ankle, put a blanket under the knees.

- Bring legs closer together if there is pain in the hamstrings and a pulling behind the knee is too much.

Meridians: Urinary bladder, stomach and spleen meridians, kidney and gallbladder

FROG/DEEP CHILD'S POSE

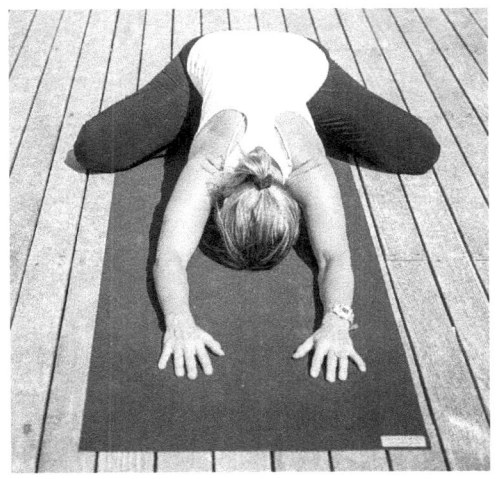

Pose: Start in Child's Pose and bring knees outside, point toes back, hands coming forward and slide down with chest. To get out, slide hands slowly back again, bring chest up, and pull knees back into Child's Pose. Stay here or lay down prone with legs together

Target area: Hips, deep groin opener (attention adductors), lower back (compression and slight back bend) and shoulders, helps for menstrual cramps and digestion

Options:

• You can also bring heels outside so that they are in line with knees (full frog).

• Lift hips higher so they are also in line with knees.

• Only one arm forward, other arm under head, change sides.

• Rest with chest on a bolster to relax upper body.

- Spread arms and hands wide if shoulders are tight.

Contraindications:

- Careful with back problems.

- With neck problems (like stiffness), rest on forehead to relax neck or stay on bolster with chest.

- Stiff shoulder, keep arms apart.

Meridians: Spleen meridians (inner knees), liver and kidney (inner groins), heart and lung meridians (with arms stretched forward)

HAPPY BABY

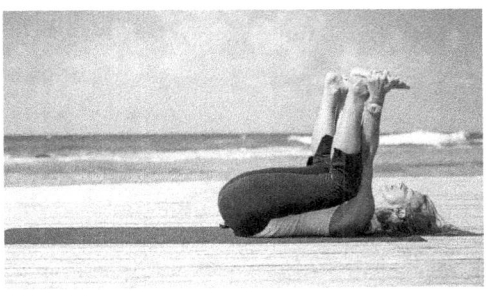

Pose: Lay on back, bend your knees toward the chest, have your arms inside of the knees and grab your feet with hands from the outside of the foot. With hands, pull your knees down toward the chest alongside of the body, keep shoulder blades down and neck relaxed. To come out of the pose, slowly relax legs down, feet on the floor and pause, then lengthen one leg after the other on the floor and stretch body.

Target area: Hips, groins, SI joints (sacroiliac joints), lumbar region.

Options:

- If you are very tight, just do one side after the other, and/or use a strap around the foot.

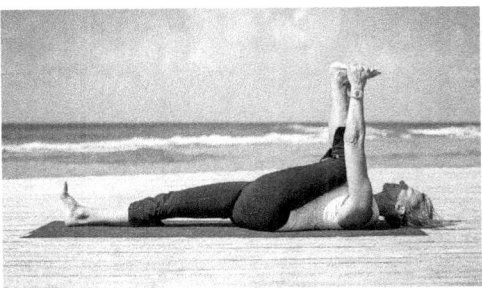

- With both legs up, change the position of the tailbone, once down forward, it will open behind the lumbar spine; once tailbone comes up and lumbar spine down (release of SI joint here), feel the difference.

Contraindications:

- With problems in SI joint, do not pull your feet down too much.

- With lower back problems, do not let hip roll up so that spine goes into flexion.

Meridians: Liver and kidney (through inner groins), urinary bladder and spine stimulation

RECLINING TWIST

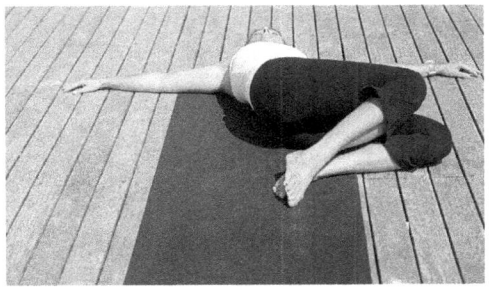

Pose: Lay on back, knees bent, feet close to hips, arms wide out to the side on shoulder level, bring knees slowly down to one side, look over to the other side (or keep looking toward ceiling). To come out, bring knees up toward the ceiling and hug knees a moment to release sacrum and lumbar spine. If done at the end of the practice, you can stay in savasana.

Target area: If knees are low, the lumbar spine/sacrum is affected); if knees are higher toward the chest, the twist will be felt higher up in spine, massages stomach organs and cures gastritis, tissue in upper chest, around shoulder and breast are stretched; pose done at the end of the practice bring equilibrium into nervous system and releases tension in the spine

Options:

- Change the position of the head, either look up toward ceiling or to opposite side of knees.

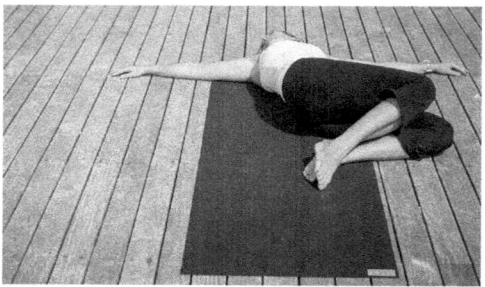

- Position of arms can also be higher over the head or next to shoulder; if shoulder blade is coming up, use blanket under that area.

- Lengthen the upper leg over to the hand (maybe hold foot with hand). This gives more a stretch than a twist.

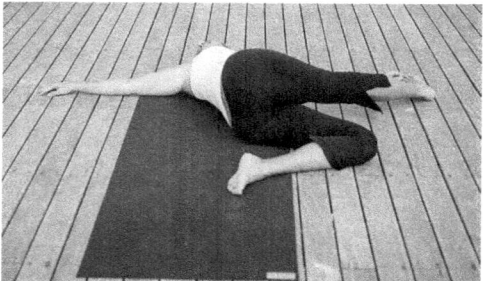

- For deeper opening in the lumbar region put the foot of the lower leg on the upper knee. Try to have both shoulder blades on the floor, otherwise use blanket behind shoulder that is floating. See what position is good for your head and neck (looking toward ceiling or either side).

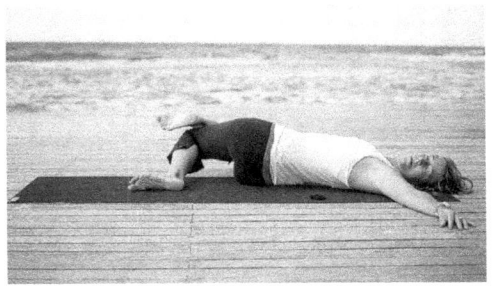

Contraindications:

- With shoulder issues (rotator cuff injuries), you might feel tingling in arms/hands. In this case, keep arm bend on ribcage or rest on a bolster.

Meridians: Urinary bladder through twisting spine, gallbladder through twisting rib cage, if one arm is overhead, heart, lung, small and large intestines are stimulated

SADDLE

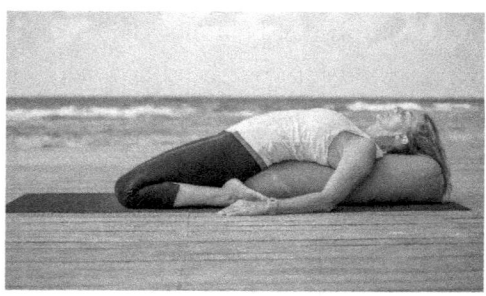

Pose: Sit down for Child's Pose and have feet pointed back outside of hips on the floor. If you already feel stress in your knees, this pose might be too much (do Sphinx or Cat Pulling Its Tail). Otherwise, go back with the spine and bring elbows on floor, touching your feet with your hands.

Target area: Abdominal organs and pelvic region, stretch in thigh and hip flexors

Options:

- Sphinx pose can be an option. Do not force yourself into saddle.

- Only bend one leg back to the side, other straight forward on the floor.

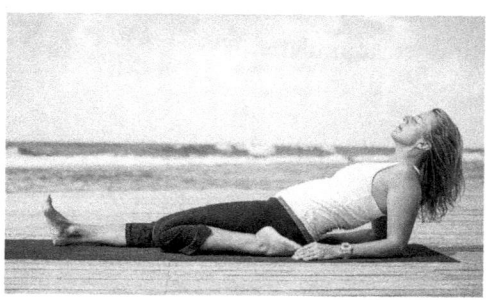

- Rest with back on a long bolster, bend one knee to the side, the other leg stays up in front with bent knee and foot on the floor.

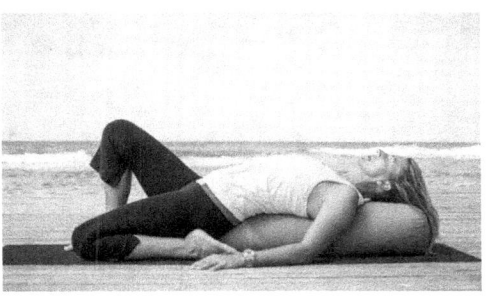

Contraindications:

- With bad back or tight sacroiliac (SI) joints, avoid pose.

- Careful with knee problems.

- Choose a variation to avoid ankle pain.

Meridians: Urinary bladder through twisting spine, gallbladder through twisting rib cage, if one arm is overhead, heart, lung, small and large intestines are stimulated

SHOELACE

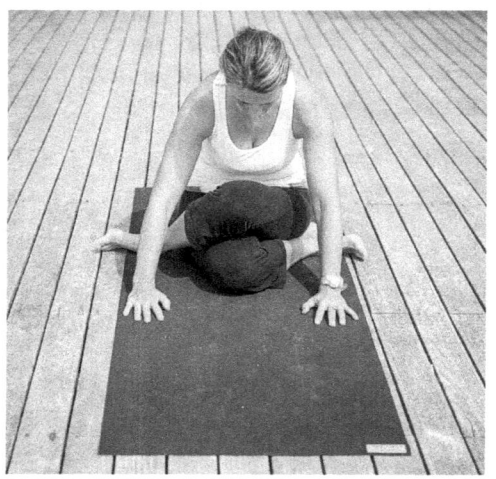

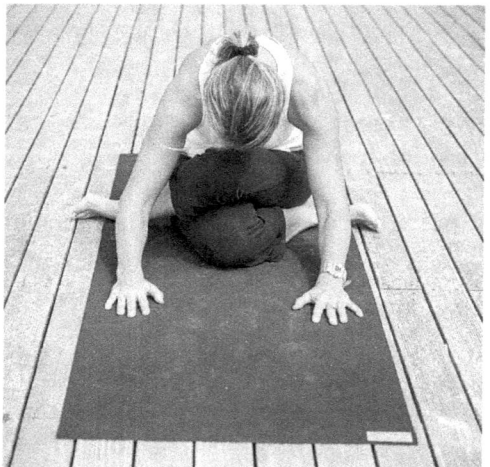

Pose: There are different ways to get into this pose. One is to go on all fours and place one knee in front of the other, spread the heels out and sit back in between the heels, do not sit on heels or foot. You should have one foot on each side outside of hip (right foot outside of left hip, left foot outside of right hip). One knee is over the other. If you feel pain or stress in bottom knee, just keep bottom leg straight forward.

If you feel pain or stress in upper leg, use bolster or blanket under the upper leg. Sit straight or slowly bend over with the chest, round the spine, hands relaxed on the floor next to legs. If there is too much stress on the outside of the hip, do not bend forward, just sit straight. To get out of the pose, slowly lift the upper leg and then lengthen; same with other side. Repeat other side starting on all fours.

Target area: Hips and lower spine

Options:

- Head can be supported on a bolster, in hands or block.

- Position of arms can vary—just relax them at side or behind the back.

- The lower leg stays forward, only upper knee is bent over lower knee.

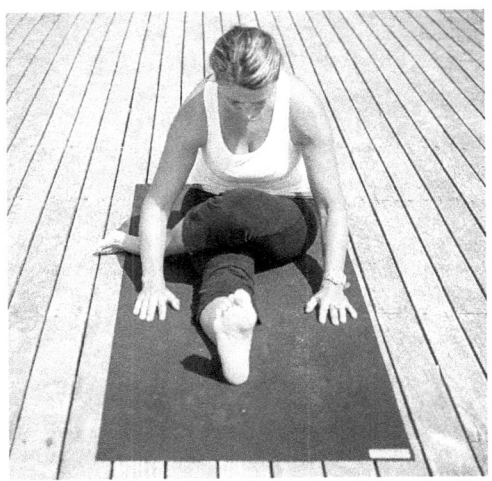

- Straight spine or spine curved forward, belly button in, shoulder blades back and down.

- Side twist with upper body can be added.

Contraindications:

- With shoulder issues (rotator cuff injuries), you might feel tingling in arms/hands. In this case, keep arm bent on ribcage or rest on a bolster.

Meridians: Liver, kidney, gallbladder; with forward fold of chest, urinary bladder and stomach organs (compressed)

SNAIL

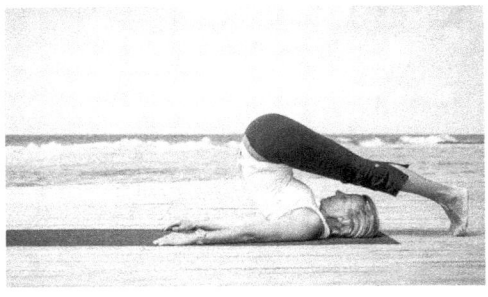

Pose: Lay on back, bend your knees towards your chest, lengthen legs up toward the ceiling, you can use abdominal strength and pressure of hands into the floor to bring legs over the head, down to the floor, spine can be rounded. Avoid pressure on the neck (some will be okay), but weight should be more onto your shoulders. To come out, the easiest way is to bend the knees, and slowly roll down with the spine until sacrum is on the floor, you can hold your legs with your hands. Hug your knees for a moment to release behind the lumbar spine, put feet on the mat for some breaths, then lengthen one leg after the other onto the mat.

Target area: The whole spine, internal organs

Options:

- Support the back with your hands, elbows on the floor can be an easier version of this pose.

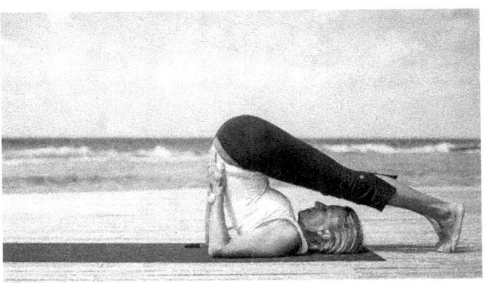

111

- Spine is round and legs over the body, bend knees so that they are coming down next to the ears.

- Option to come out of the pose: With long legs (demands more abdominal strength).

Contraindications:

- With neck problems, do not fold over as it puts a lot of pressure on the neck.

- Not recommended with high blood pressure, upper body infection, glaucoma, or cold.

- When menstruating, you may want to avoid this pose.

- With lower back problems, you might want to avoid flexion in that region of the spine.

- With shoulder blade problems, you do not want to bring hands together on the floor, keep arms straight and outside of body.

Meridians: Deep stretch for urinary bladder, all stomach organs compressed; with breaths, the massage of organs can be deepened

SUPTA PADANGUSTHASANA

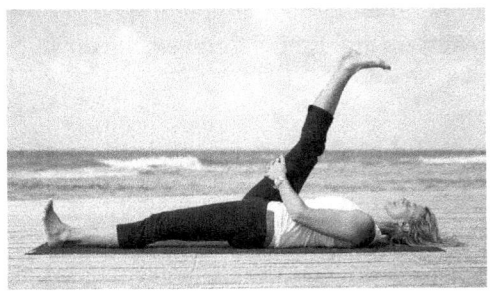

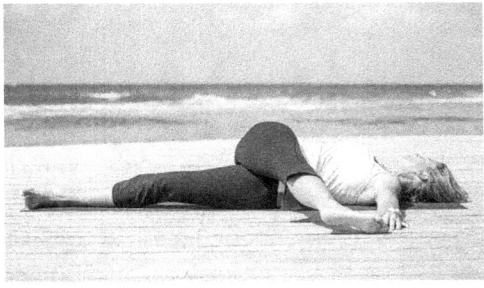

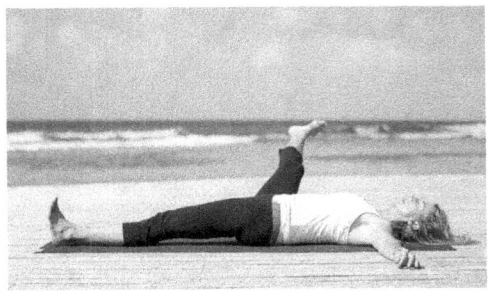

Pose: Lay supine, bend one knee toward the chest and then straighten up toward the ceiling. With hands, clasp behind the thigh while keeping the back in neutral. Let gravity work and the weight of the leg will come down in the hip, relax leg muscles and foot. The other leg stays straight on the floor, pressing into the ground. After a while, bring the upper leg down to the side. When going down to the right with the right leg, keep left hip down. When going down to the left with the right leg, keep hips over each other. To come out of the pose, have the leg straight up and then bend it slowly down and lengthen on the floor.

Target area: Back of the thigh, leg, and sacrum

Options:

- Use a strap around the foot to lengthen the leg up toward the ceiling.

Contraindication:

- Avoid the variation with the leg to the side if you have SI joint problems or herniated disc; just do straight leg variation.

SPHINX / SEAL

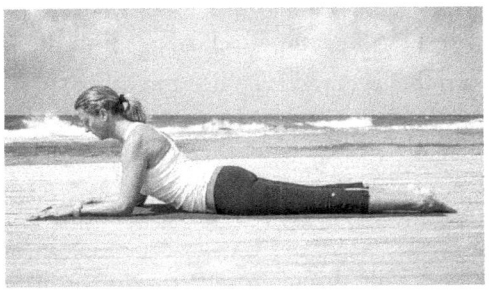

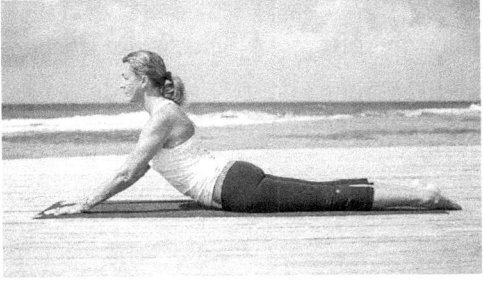

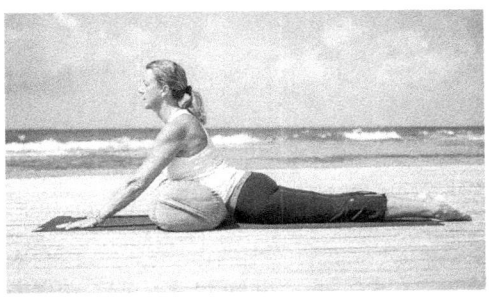

Pose: Lay down, prone, bring elbows under the shoulder and forearm long forward, see how it feels. If there is pinching or pressure in lower back (especially L2/L3 region), walk your elbows a bit forward of the shoulders and lower the chest. The more pressure or pinching you feel in your lower back, the more you can walk forward and lower chest being in a low Sphinx pose or completely prone on the floor. To come out, you slowly lower the chest and rest your forefront on hands, or you turn your head to one side and you pull the knee on the same side up next to the chest (still prone, it relaxes behind the lumber region), then you lengthen the leg back, turn head to other side, and pull up the other knee toward your other side of the chest.

Target area: Lower spine (lumbar region) and neck/cervical spine area when neck is back

Options:

- Bring forearms on bolster or blocks, which deepens the pose behind the lumbar spine.

- Decide for yourself the safest arm position to avoid sharp pain behind lumbar spine.

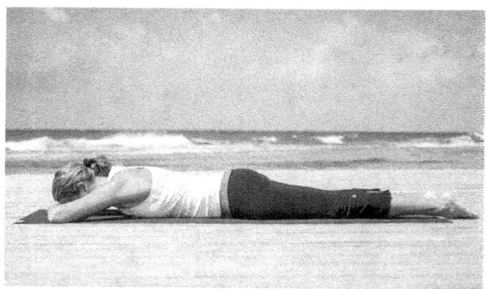

- According to Paulie Zink, you can have arms straight out to the side, which makes it more a seal pose.

- Feel if you prefer legs long and together to have release in sacrum. The effect is more along the spine.

- If too much pressure under pubic bone, use blanket. If pregnant, use bolster.

- You can stimulate the neck and cervical spine by lengthening the neck and lifting chin up.

Contraindication:

- With neck problems, do not fold over as it puts a lot of pressure on the neck.

Meridians: Urinary bladder, kidney, stomach and spleen; With more compression, adrenal glands stimulated with kidneys

SQUARE

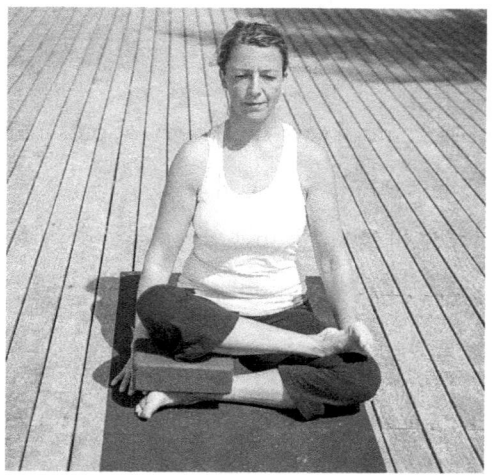

Pose: Sit with straight spine and legs crossed, then bring your shins forward so that they are parallel with the mat (which might be already difficult!), bring one shin on top of the other so that one knee is over the opposite ankle. Be careful here because if the hips are too tight, the pressure transfers into the knees, and that's what you should avoid. To come out, lean slightly back and lengthen your legs forward; repeat on other side.

Target area: Hips and spine

Options:

- You might want to use a block between the knee and the foot if there is a big gap.

- You can fold forward and even lengthen arms forward if your hips allow it. I recommend sitting on a blanket or cushion for this; the stretch will be deeper in lower back.

- If hips are too tight, use a bolster so that knees are lower than hips.

Contraindications:

- Avoid pose with sciatica problems as it can aggravate it.

- Be aware of hips. If too tight, they might rotate backward, but they should stay forward.

Meridians: Urinary bladder, kidney, stomach and spleen; with more compression, adrenal glands stimulated with kidneys

Other Variations:

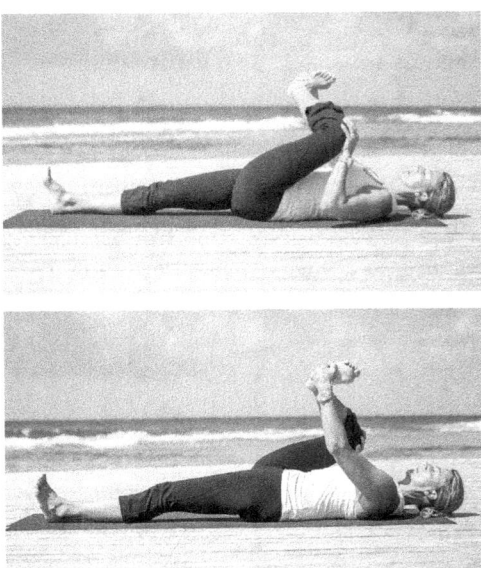

SQUAT

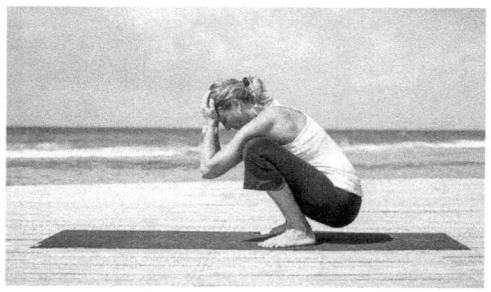

Pose: Stand with feet wider than hip distance apart and toes pointing out, hands in prayer (anjali mudra), then bend knees and sit down, elbows come in between the knees, forearms on one straight line. You can slightly press with elbows against knees and knees against elbows, which brings more sensation into hip area. Let the tailbone drop down. Hands can also come down in front of you. If heels are up and not coming down on floor, use a blanket under heels or widen the feet. Knees should point in same direction as feet. Easily come down, slowly sit back down, and lengthen legs out to the front. A more difficult version to come out, as it demands strength in the legs, is pushing feet into floor to bring hips up and folding chest forward into Dangling Pose.

Target area: Hips, knees and ankles, lower back

Options:

• With feet close together, the pose works deeper on the ankle.

• With feet hip distance apart or a bit wider, it works more in the hip.

• A more advanced version of the pose is with feet together but knees apart, folding forward and bringing arms around the shins to the back with clasping hands.

Contraindications:

- Avoid if you have had knee trauma.

- Tight hips can play a role in your knees, so be careful.

Meridians: Urinary bladder, kidney, and liver; through ankle, you can stimulate stomach, spleen, gallbladder and urinary bladder

Other Variations:

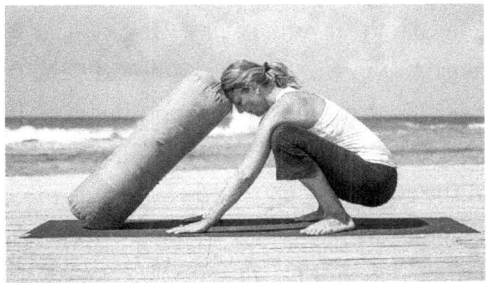

SWAN

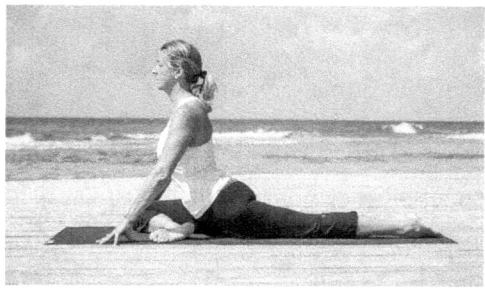

Pose: Coming from Downward Facing Dog or Cat Pose, bring one knee forward close to the wrist on the same side, the foot comes over to the opposite side, foot can be under opposite groin or further to the front, that brings more pressure in the hip. Stay parallel in hips, avoid falling down on the butt, only come down if knee, hip and foot allows it. Otherwise, use bolster, cushion, or blanket under butt side. If knee is fine, flex ankle and bring foot further forward. Stay here with chest up, Swan can be a gentle back bend, but if you are more flexible it can go deeper into the back bend while bringing your arms over your head or clasping hands behind the back and opening even the chest area. This sounds more like the yang Pigeon Pose, but your joints are still in yin. You can also bring the back leg bending with the heel toward the butt so the stretch in your thigh gets much deeper. Always listen to your body and stay connected with your hips and knees. Be gentle.

Target area: Hips, knees and ankles; lower back when folding forward

Options:

- You might want to use a block between the knee and the foot if there is a big gap.

- You can fold forward and even lengthen arms forward if your hips allow it; the stretch will be deeper in lower back then. I recommend sitting on a blanket or cushion for this.

- If hips are too tight, sit on a bolster so that knees are lower than hips.

Contraindication:

- Avoid if you have had knee trauma.

Meridians: Urinary bladder, kidney, and liver; through ankle, you can stimulate stomach, spleen, gallbladder and urinary bladder

Other Variations:

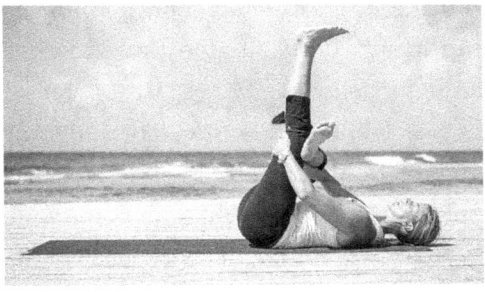

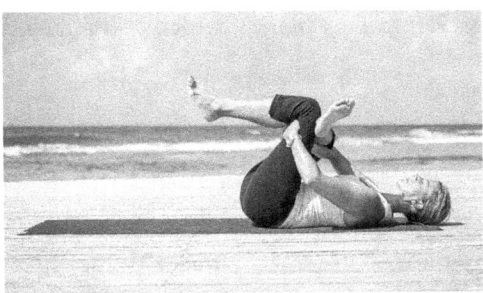

SLEEPING SWAN

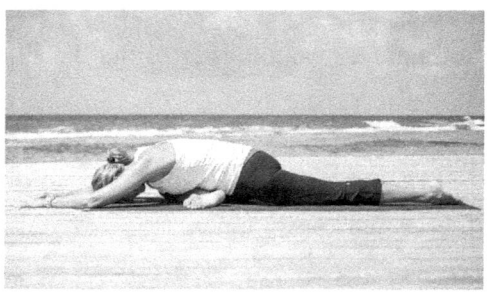

Pose: From Down Dog, bring one knee forward close to the wrist on the same side, the foot comes over to the opposite side, foot can be under opposite groin or further to the front, that brings more pressure in the hip. Stay parallel in hips, avoid falling down on the butt, only come down if knee, hip and foot allows it. Otherwise, use bolster, cushion or blanket under butt side. If knee is fine, flex ankle and bring foot further forward. Depending on your hips and knee, come further down on forearms, or lay on a bolster with the chest, or come completely down with chest onto the mat. To come out of pose, push your hands into the mat to bring the chest up, tuck your toes on back foot under and push the hip area up back into Down Dog, which will feel great now. Walk your legs out.

Target area: Hips, lower back (especially in full swan)

Options:

• With block or blanket under the hip side of the leg, which is in the front.

• Laying down with chest on bolster or completely down on mat.

• If you stay up with the chest, almost slightly in a back bend (compressing lower back), it is a full swan and the weight is completely going into the hip as the weight is placed above it (allow gravity to do the work).

Contraindications:

- Knee trauma, meniscus etc., watch pressure in knee.

- Hip pain. A lot of pressure in hip if hips are very tight, then bring foot further toward the groin.

Meridians: Kidney, liver, stomach, spleen, gallbladder and urinary bladder

VIPARITA KARANI

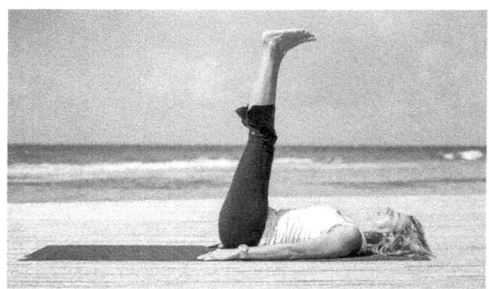

Pose: Sit with your hip side against the wall, knees bent, and feet on the floor, while turning to the wall, swing both legs up and lay down on back, legs and torso are in 90-degree angle, you are facing the ceiling. Keep your arms on the floor, shoulder blades relaxed down, legs straight up. Having a small weight (like a cushion) on the top of your feet increases the relaxing effect. Keep your eyes closed and just surrender. Stay focused on the breath, this pose calms the nervous system and rejuvenates the circulatory system. To come out of the pose, gently bend your knees toward your chest and roll down to one side, stay here for a couple of deep breaths before you come up to a seated position.

Target area: Hamstring, lower back, nervous system, circulatory system, lymph system

Options:

- Block or blanket under the sacrum

- Hands resting on the chest or belly, long aside the ears or behind the head

- When legs start tingling, bend knees to the side and bring the feet down

- Instead of doing the pose against a wall, just bend knees and have calves resting on a chair (90 degrees angle)

- Legs against the wall is a great option during menstruation cycle to release menstrual cramps or water retention in legs

Contraindications:

- Avoid with glaucoma, after eye surgery, or high blood pressure

- With hamstring or back injuries (do chair version)

Meridians: Digestive (stomach and liver), nervous end endocrine system

Other Variations:

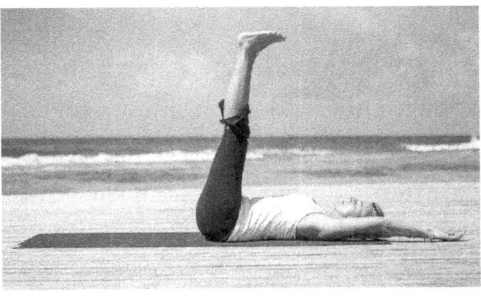

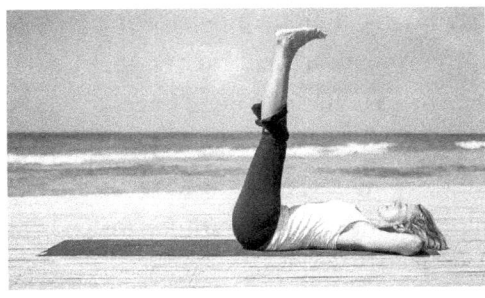

SAVASANA

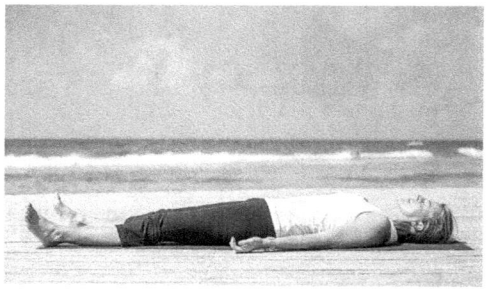

Pose: Finally, the pose to release all tension, contraction, and stuff that is going on in the mind. Just feel your body laying on the floor, let your weight melt down in the mat. This pose has the benefit of complete relaxation so that body and mind become stronger. Feel the bliss (samadhi) of this pose. After a session, you do not want to fall asleep, but recognize the changes in the body, energy that is flowing and calming down. Sometimes after a yin session, we do not need a long savasana, but do not skip it.

Maybe you finish the practice with a pose that brings you already on your back, laying down. Otherwise, from sitting with knees bent (safer for your lumbar spine), roll slowly down on your back, relax shoulders, arms on the side of your body and neck completely relaxed, lengthen legs hip distance apart or a bit wider, let feet fall to any side so that it feels comfortable for your sacrum. Close your eyes and try not to fall asleep. Scan your body for a moment, observing your breath. To get out of the pose, bring your awareness back to your body, take a breath in your belly, wiggle toes and fingers, bend knees to your chest and roll on the right side, stay there a moment before you push yourself up to a comfortable seat, keeping neck and head relaxed while coming up. Take some deep breaths and feel the gratitude for your practice, body, and mind.

Target area: Relax the whole body, mind, and spirit; calm breath

Options:

- Use bolster under your knees.

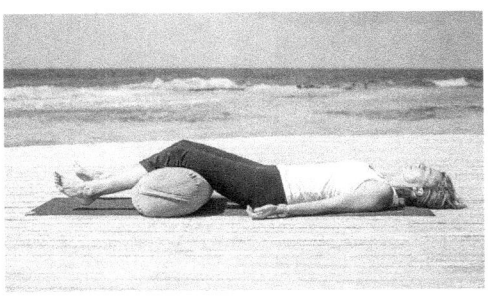

- Place a blanket under your neck.

Contraindications:

- Some people can get anxious while in savasana or deep relaxation. Observe your situation, maybe consult a doctor.

- The effects of medication can be intensified in deep relaxation.

- Repressed emotions can occur in deep relaxation. Stay focused on the breath.

YANG POSES AS COUNTERPOSES

The following is an outline of yin poses that I have chosen, but there are more if you go to LIGHT ON YOGA by BKS Iyengar. With these poses, you can begin to build your own flow.

CAT COW FLOW

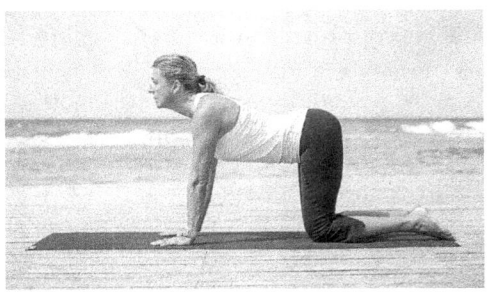

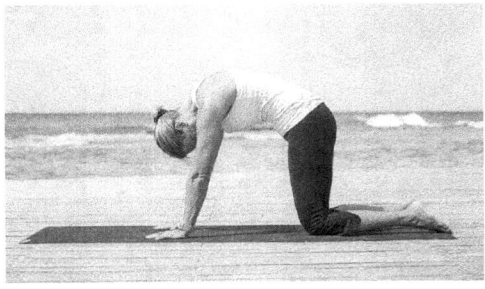

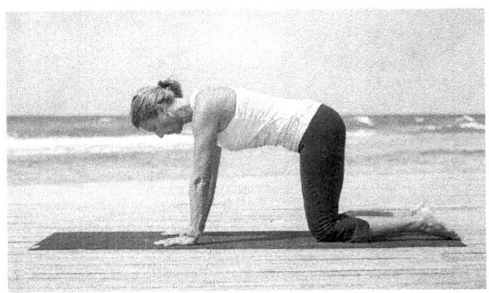

Pose: Start on all fours, wrists under shoulders, knees under hips, straight spine, take a deep inhale. With an exhale, arch your spine up toward the ceiling, head is coming forward and down (crown down to earth), tailbone going back and down, feel shoulder blades spread wide. Here, you are in Cow Pose. With an inhale, bring spine and navel down to floor, relax belly, head is going up and tail bone is going up. With next exhale, repeat the movement to bring head forward and down and tail bone back and down to Cow Pose again with a long arching spine. Repeat this for your own comfort to feel energized again.

This Cat Cow Flow is complimentary the breathing of Arowhan Awarohan, creating space in your body and focusing inside (pratjahara, inside observation).

Target area: Stretches upper part of the body like shoulders, spinal extensors, and neck; can even strengthen arms and shoulder blades

DOWNWARD FACING DOG

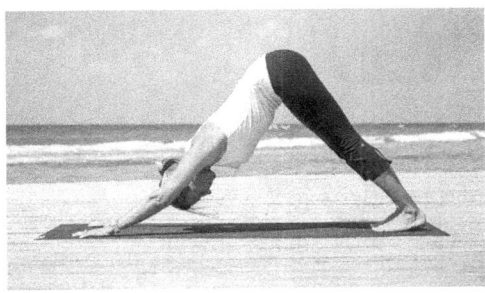

Pose: Start on all fours, bring hands slightly in front of the shoulders, spread fingers wide, press hands and toes into the mat to lift up hips and knees. With the pressure in your hands, bring chest further toward thighs and feel the stretch behind the legs.

Target area: Hamstring stretch, lengthening of both sides of torso (good for scoliosis), shoulder opener

PARS VAJRASANA / MERMAID

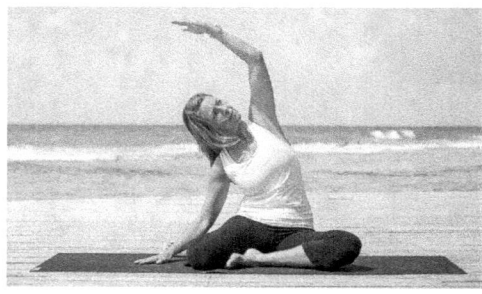

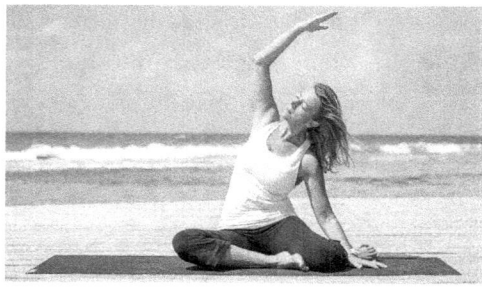

Pose: Sitting on shinbones and heels, slide down to one side to have buttocks on the floor and the bottom foot on the top ankle, or like here in the photo, just in front of the thigh, keep hips straight, bring the arm of the side where the knees are pointing to up toward the ceiling and stretch it over the head to the other side, feel the opening and lengthening of that side. To go deeper, turn the chest to the side with the arm up and even rotate slightly to look up toward the ceiling. Slowly go back into center and bring arm down. To repeat on other side, you can swing the legs and feet forward and to the other side.

Target area: Rib cage expansion, shoulder opener, stretch for scoliosis

Options:

- Knees wider so that one foot is in front of the other thigh. (see photo)

- With a rotation of the chest to the side of the feet, hands down.

Contraindications:

- Shoulder injuries

- Knee problems

- Rib cage injuries

SHALABASANA

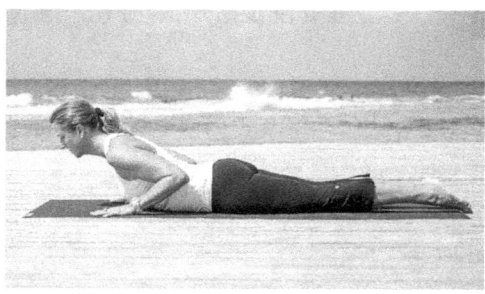

Pose: Lay long on your belly, bring hands under the shoulders, press into the mat to bring your chest up, stay for a couple of breaths. It is a nice stretch after forward fold poses, then go back into Child's Pose.

Target area: Strengthens all muscles of back and body, especially in variations where the legs come off the mat as well; with deep breathing it is opening chest and respiratory muscles, stretching diaphragm

Contraindications:

- If pregnant, do not lie prone.

- Lower back issues

SEATED TWIST

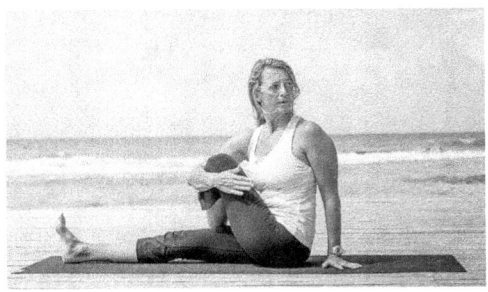

Pose: Start by sitting with legs in front of you, bend left knee and bring left foot over to the outer side of the right leg. Keep buttocks rooted, hug the left knee with the right arm and rotate to the left side, while pressing with the left hand behind your back into the mat, lengthening the spine and breathing into the ribcage. To come out of the pose, lengthen both legs in front of you , shake legs out and do the other side.

Target area: Abdominal muscles, organs for digestion, muscles along the spine (erector spinae), shoulder girdle

Other Variations:

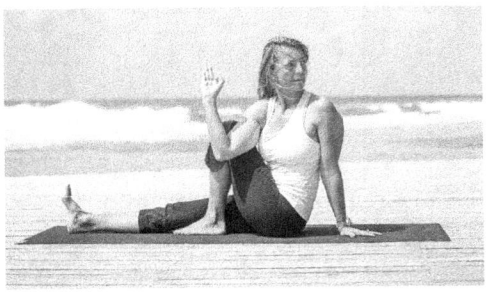

A variation can be to have the bottom knee also bend, the left foot is coming on the outside of the right hip and than the right foot is coming on the outside of the left hip. Here it is more challenging to have the buttocks rooting down and the spine straight.

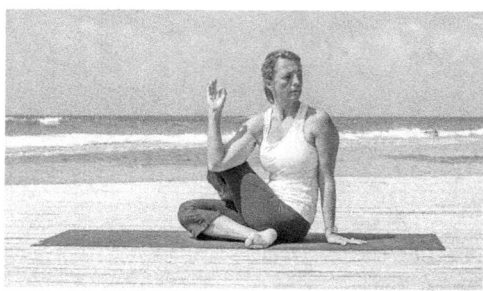

NAVASANA

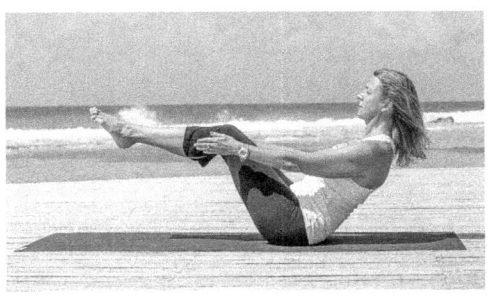

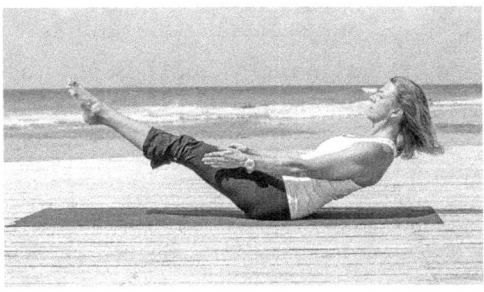

Pose: Sit straight, feet on the floor, bring your arms forward next to the knees with shoulder blades down. For a moment, just press feet into the mat to feel your abs, then bring feet on knee level with the spine straight. Do not round behind the lumbar spine, otherwise keep feet on the floor. A more challenging version is with legs straight.

Target area: Strengthening of abdominal muscles, spine muscles and hip flexors, shoulder girdle alignment, focus on breath and concentration

As you see, these yang poses are more strengthening than relaxing, but in between a yin flow, it can help you feel still and grounded.

YIN FLOW

For your own practice

FLOW 1

This is a short yin flow I like to do if I do not have a lot of time but need to wind down. It feels like a reset. You can adjust this sequence to the time you have available. If you choose three minutes per pose, it will take about 25-30 minutes total, depending on how much time you want to spend in Savasana at the end. I usually do four minutes in each pose and it takes about 35-40 minutes. Feel free to adjust to your personal needs.

Pose 1 – Sukhasana

Sit crossed legged, straight spine, hands on your knees, chin slightly to the chest. Concentrate on breathing with the Arowahn Awarohan technique, the figure eight breathing, and feel the energy moving in your body. Stay for 4-5 minutes.

Pose 2 – Sukhasana (with rotation)

Bring your hands to the ceiling, inhale. Upon exhale, rotate to the right side, stay straight with your pine, focus on breathing, stay for 2-3 minutes. Take a long inhale, bring arms up toward the ceiling, and rotate back to the center, and with exhale rotate, to the left, stay for 2-3 minutes.

Pose 3 – Butterfly

From the center, fold forward with the spine toward the floor, hands can rest on your feet or on the floor. If necessary, sit on a blanket.

Pose 4 – Bananasana

Lay on your back, bring both feet and legs touching to the right side, and with your right hand grab the left wrist to bring also the upper body and arms over to the right, keep butt and shoulder blades on the floor, focus on breathing into the ribcage, especially into the left side, create space, stay for 3-4 minutes, then slowly come back to center, stretch your body lengthwise, and change to the left side with feet and arms, now breathe into the right side of the rib cage.

Pose 5 – Cat Pulling Its Tail

Start by laying on the right side, you can have your head resting on your right arm, right leg stays straight while the left leg is coming to the right side with the knee bent. Now also bend the right knee, grab your ankle and "pull" your heel toward your buttock, feel the stretch in the right quadriceps, use the breath in this area. Keep the right hip on the floor, by rolling further to the right side you can change the pull in the quadriceps, take time to enter into the stretch. Then slowly roll back on your back and repeat on the left side, right knee is coming over and grab the left ankle to pull the left heel up to your buttock. Enjoy each side for 3-4 minutes.

Pose 6 – Bridge

Come back on your spine after Pose 5, pull both legs, spine and arms long (feet away from your hands) and take a deep breath, then bring both knees bent toward your chest, hug them and take some deep breaths. Bring feet on the floor with knees bent, hip distance apart, heels close to your butt, push your feet into the mat to lift up with your hips, just stay for a few breaths, you can bring arms behind the back on the floor with hands clasped. Stay up with your hips for a couple of deep breaths. Slowly roll the spine down, and again, bring the knees up toward your chest, hug them while you take some deep relaxing breaths.

Pose 7 – Savasana

Lengthen your whole body on the mat in Savasana. If needed, prop your body with a blanket under the knees, an eye pillow on your eyes. Rest and relax, allow your body to heal and your mind to wind down.

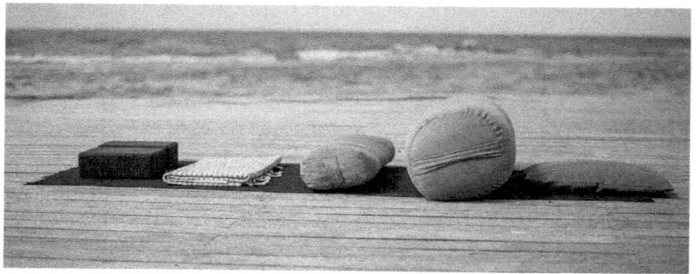

FLOW 2

This is a flow which stimulates all your organs (kidneys, urinary bladder, liver, also stomach and spleen). This flow advocates digestion, your metabolism, and releases negative emotions. It can be done in 45-60 minutes, but you decide what feels good for you. I recommend holding the poses for 4 minutes to allow the fascia to let go of the stress created by negative memories and emotions (which bring tension into the fascia).

Pose 1 – Child's Pose

Allow yourself to take time arriving on the mat. Child's Pose is a very healing and restful pose. Come in contact with your breathing, and take time to observe where you feel the breathing and what emotions are coming up. Do not judge or get attached.

Pose 2 – Downward Facing Dog

Come up out of Child's Pose to Downward Facing Dog, and stretch your legs out, take some deep breaths and stretch your whole body before you go back down on all fours to change over and lay on your back.

Pose 3 – Half Happy Baby

Bend your right leg toward your chest and pull the knee down to the right side of your chest, hands on your knees. Take awareness of your breathing in the belly and into the chest, and take time to pull with your hands down toward the chest. After 2 minutes, bring your right foot over the knee, the knee stays close to your chest. Grab your foot with your hands or use a strap or towel around the foot. Now, feel the stretch behind your hamstrings, send your breath into that area and feel what is happening, what emotion wants to come up and out. Just feel, do not judge. After 3-4 minutes, bend your knee slowly and relax your right leg slowly down to the mat. Stretch both legs long and observe the difference of the sensation you have now between right and left hip as well as right and left leg. Repeat with left leg.

Pose 4 – Tadagasana

Lay on your back with long legs and long arms stretched over your head, press your heels, legs, and back elbows into the mat and feel the length of your whole body on the floor; create length between feet and hands. Now, breathe into the rib cage, feel your belly like a pond and use the breathing in your diaphragm where we hold a lot of emotion and tension.

Pose 5 – Dragonfly

Come into seated position. I recommend using a blanket under your seat, spread your legs wide apart (see what's comfortable for you). If you have knee problems, also use a blanket under your knees or bend knees slightly. Sit with your spine straight and slowly roll forward—that gives you a stretch behind the lower back and behind the legs, in the groin and inner thighs. Breathe slowly and deeply and get in touch with the area where you feel the stretch. With time, the areas where you feel the stretch might change to around the hips or behind the back. Maybe you will feel it even in your face. Stay connected and relax into the pose. Gently come out of the pose after 4 minutes, slowly bring your legs close together and shake them out.

Pose 6 – Shoelace

Keep your left leg straight and bend the right knee over, the right foot is coming next to your outer left hip. If possible, now bend the left knee so that the left foot is coming outside of the right hip. If this is too much, as your hips are too tight, stay with the left leg long. To intensify the stretch, come toward your knees with your spine and neck forming an arch. This will intensify the stretch behind the lower back and outside of your hips. After 3-4 minutes, change sides, taking your time to do so. After the pose, slowly come over on all fours for a counter position.

Pose 7 – Cat Cow Sequence

Have your wrist under the shoulders and knees under the hips. Circle with your hips around the knees and do 3-4 movements of cat cow. This is to bring some movements in the joints and energy flowing.

Pose 8 – Sphinx/Seal

Lay down, prone, hipbones and legs are on the floor, elbows under your shoulders, shoulder blades away from the ears and forearms parallel. Bring length into the spine and neck. You can vary the position of your elbows, move them maybe slightly in front of the shoulders if this is still comfortable for your lower back. Let go of tension/contraction in lower back and buttocks, have the legs relaxed on the mat. You can also use a cushion under your forearms if it is possible for you to bring your chest higher up, which will increase the stimulation of the sacral lumbar arch. If this is too much, just lay down, prone, with your elbows bent and the arms used like a cushion under your head. Relax and breathe. Slowly bring yourself back into Child's Pose as a counter pose.

Pose 9 – Child's Pose

Keep your buttocks back on your heels and find your breath in your ribcage. Stay focused on the breath and relax the mind.

Pose 10 – Savasana

Sit down and slowly roll your spine back while your knees are bent and your feet on the floor. Then, lengthen your legs in front of you, hip distance apart, let them fall outside. If necessary, use a bolster or blanket behind your knees. Let your shoulder blades relax onto the floor, the arms are resting comfortably away from the body. If you want to use a blanket on your body to support the resting mode of your nervous system, feel free to do so. Savasana represents the end of your yin flow, so take time to heal and complete the sequence. Stay relaxed and pay attention to the changes you created in your body energetically, physically, and mentally.

The more you practice, the more you will notice energies and feelings. It will also increase your awareness not only in your yoga practice, but also in your daily life, which will help you to become more mindful, with the goal to become happier and healthier. The more you are connected with your body and mind, the better decisions you can make for your life. Go for your desire and live it. Get out of fear and into the vibration of love, which is the highest and healthiest vibration we have. Do not settle for less. You are worthy of happiness, greatness, love, and respect.

"Only when our clever brain and human hearts work together in harmony can we achieve our true potential."

-Jane Goodall

Conclusion

My purpose in writing this book was not only to give you a little more insight into how yin and yang philosophy can be integrated into your life and health, but to also help you deeply investigate your own way of living, your thoughts, your connection to others, and your relationship to food, work, and exercise. You have the power to make changes and to heal. You can empower yourself, take your life into your own hands, and know there are ways to make positive change. Change might eventually require some courage, but first, it needs some awareness and consciousness in your life. When you bring awareness to a situation in which you are not comfortable or happy with, you get the chance to evolve and change it.

If something feels wrong in your body or you feel sick, it does not necessarily mean that there is something physically wrong with your body. We forget that we also have a spiritual body, and if we ignore our spiritual bodies, problems might manifest in our physical bodies. All of the pain I experienced over the years was never related to a real medical problem. Even my toothaches, which had me at the dentist once a month, were not caused by a real dental problem, like gum disease or periodontitis. It was stress and grinding my teeth at night. By just healing the symptom, it never stopped hurting. Eventually, we all have to learn how to address the cause, not just the symptom.

I faked happiness for many years of my life. I thought that I should be happy with what I had, that I should be grateful. But there is a difference between real happiness in your heart and artificial happiness.

When we are unhappy, we become used to the thought that something is wrong with us, and we might even feel ungrateful for what we have or feel guilty if we feel sad. We start feeling confused, angry even, and it can be easy to start spreading our unhappiness around. In the worst case, we may even blame others for our feelings and unhappiness. The key to finding balance and happiness is inside all of us, but to get there, we need to become aware of our situation and take responsibility for our feelings. We need to be brave.

Once you become aware of the things you want to change, I've offered you some ideas about where you can start making little changes, because little changes often lead to even bigger changes for a happier and healthier life.

Once I understood that I should not suffer, that I have the right to live without suffering, that I should not have to fight for everything, I realized that there must be a way to have an easier life. Life should not be full of obstacles or misunderstandings, it should not be painful to go to our jobs or participate in our relationships, and our food shouldn't make us sick. If this is the case, there is something wrong. If you are not happy in your relationship, there is something wrong. If you are going to a job every morning which you do not like, there is something wrong. And if you are unhappy but think everything is the way it should be, there is really something wrong. Pain is like a teacher. It shows the way to something better. It is the path of unbecoming so that you may build yourself back up into the person you desire to be with the life you deserve to have.

Despite what you might think, life changes should be simple. There is nothing extraordinary to leading a great life. The hardest thing about making life changes is accepting that we have the right to pursue them. We spend so much time trying to please other people and their perceptions of us that we create distance from our true Self. This cycle is what leads to unhappiness, sickness, and depression, which are signs from the Universe to help you to understand that change is needed.

Change begins with a first step, which might be a tiny step. Little changes in the way you nurture yourself can quickly bring more balance into your life. Changes in the way you frame your thoughts can have a big impact because our thoughts become our beliefs, and our beliefs become our habits, and our habits become our truth, a false truth. Start by focusing on changing just your thoughts and the rest will follow.

Becoming aware of stagnant patterns in our lives often creates fear. Let go of the fear of change. Though fear can be a giant obstacle that holds us back, fear is more a thought than a real thing. It is something we create in a situation that went wrong, and we start thinking things are unchangeable. You were bitten by a dog once and now you fear all dogs, but not all dogs will bite you. So the fear is created by just one situation in which you suffered, and now to avoid that same suffering, you avoid all dogs. Another common example of this in when we get hurt in relationships. We get hurt so we avoid falling in love again, not another breakup. Being hurt once does not mean that it will always happen, but we create the fear of being hurt and try to avoid it.

By being in a situation you do not like, like a job or a relationship, you suffer. To protect yourself from feeling the pain of financial stress or another breakup, you stay at your job or in a bad relationship. Because we are used to this feeling and have learned how to deal with it, we stay close to what we know—suffering. What we know, even if it's negative, gives us a feeling of safety. We master our situations, and we even master our pain.

When you start to change, it is not just you who will benefit. You become an example for others. Through you, others might start to reflect on their life, become more aware, and feel inspired to also make improvements in their life. The more happy people we have, the more we can influence the environment. It's a ripple effect that will improve the people around you, they will improve people around them, and so on, increasing the energy and vibration in the universe. Change is an opportunity for growth and openness. It means letting go of the old and being open to something new. I've never, ever met somebody who regretted a change. It is always an improvement, even if the transition from one life story to another is not easy. Change is the path to freedom.

Balance is the most important element to living a healthy life in a healthy body. Being out of balance means we are putting our body under stress, not valuing ourselves, and increasing the chance of attracting disease. Become aware. As soon as you understand what's going on, you have the chance to change. If I was able to change, you can change too. I wish you all the courage and bravery needed to take a leap and live the awesome life you have always dreamed of.

> *"Fight your fears and you'll be in battle forever.*
> *Face your fears, and you'll be free forever."*
>
> -Lucas Jonkman

Recommended Readings

Yin Yoga: An Individualized Approach to Balance, Health and Whole Well-Being by Ulrica Norberg

The Complete Guide to Yin Yoga by Bernie Clark

Inside Yoga by Sarah Powers

Light on Yoga by Iyengar

About The Author

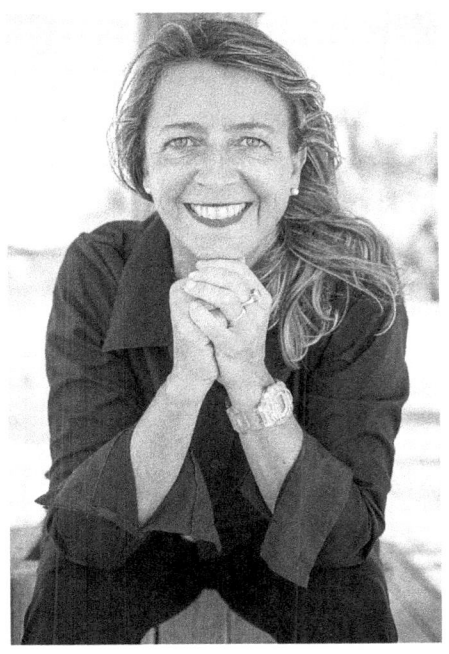

Petra Rakebrandt is a Holistic Life Coach in Guadeloupe. After completing her studies for civil engineering and a MBA, Petra found herself indifferent about her chosen profession. Despite her reservations, it felt right and safe initially, but overtime, discontentment grew. She always dreamed of a different life that did not follow mainstream expectations and pace. After challenges at work and in marriage, her feelings of disconnect between her personal desires and current reality led her to experience sickness and a loss of connection to herself. Rising from the darkness, Petra realized her true passion for healing and the healing arts, and seeks to bring empathy and understanding to all she impacts. Clients, friends, and family know her for her empathy, strong intuition, and sensitivity. Her path to this book began with her discovery of yoga and meditation. Petra brings a ten-year background with healing modalities and studies in nutrition from the Institute for Integrative Nutrition, certification as a yoga instructor through Yogiraj, Alan Finger, Ishta Yoga NYC, Stott Pilates instructor and personal fitness coach. Petra is known internationally for her work, and she strives to incorporate skill development and education into her international retreats.

"By healing the soul, we can improve our health and happiness, and give our bodies the chance to self-heal so that we can support friends and family, and work to make the Universe a better place."

-Petra Rakebrandt

Notes

MY IMBALANCES:

Notes

MY FIRST LITTLE STEPS OF CHANGE:

Notes

MY OWN CREATED YIN FLOW:

Notes

Notes

Notes

Notes

Notes

Notes

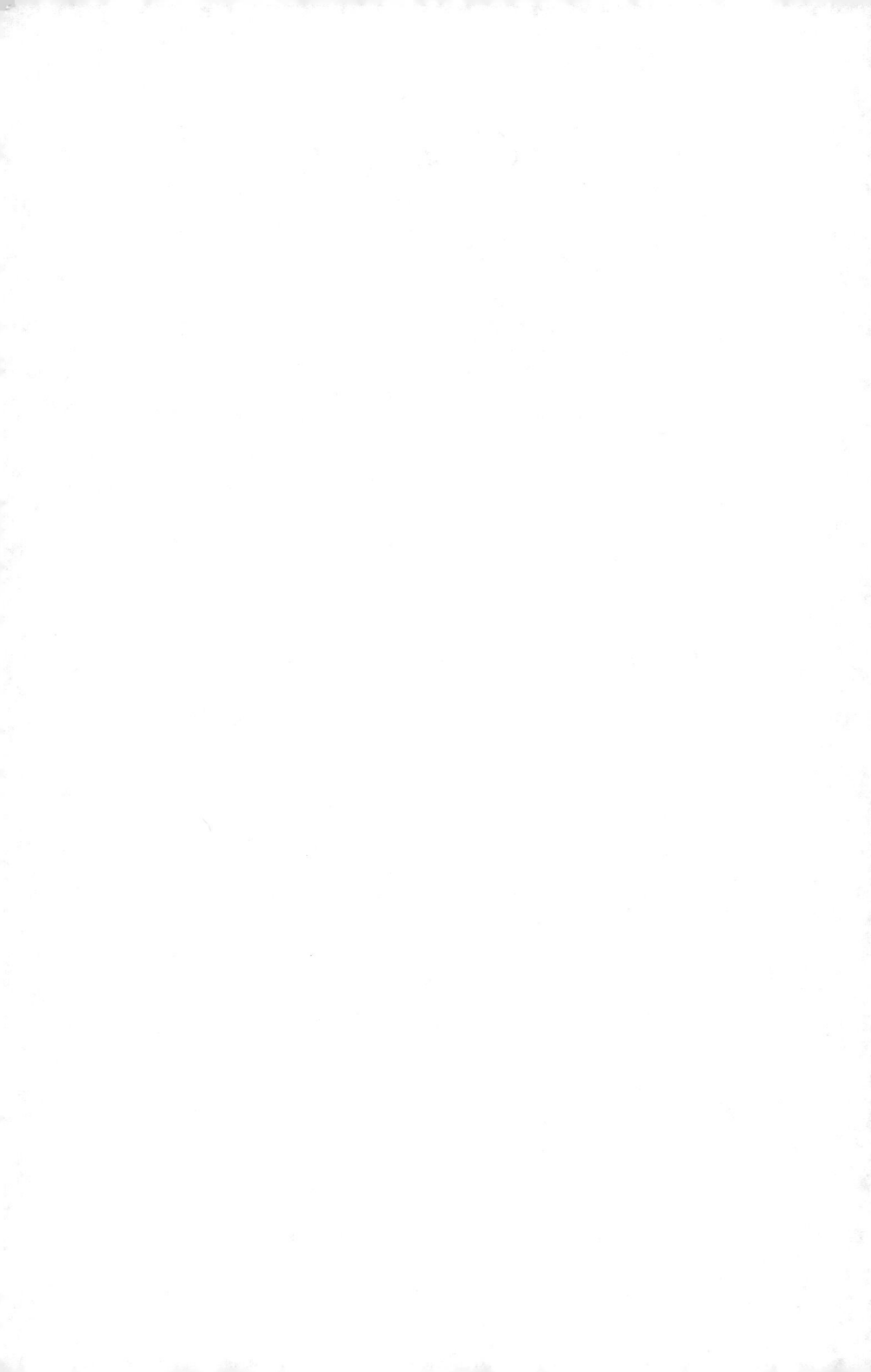